100 Questions & Answers About Your Child's Depression or Bipolar Disorder

Linda Chokroverty, MD, FAAP

Assistant Clinical Professor
Departments of Psychiatry
and Behavioral Sciences and Pediatrics
Albert Einstein College of Medicine of Yeshiva University
Bronx, NY
and
Child and Adolescent Psychiatrist
Director, Outpatient Pediatrics
The Bronx Children's Psychiatric Center
Day Treatment Program
Bronx, NY

JONES AND BARTLETT PUBLISHERS
Sudbury, Massachusetts
BOSTON   TORONTO   LONDON   SINGAPORE

World Headquarters
Jones and Bartlett Publishers
40 Tall Pine Drive
Sudbury, MA 01776
978-443-5000
info@jbpub.com
www.jbpub.com

Jones and Bartlett Publishers
Canada
6339 Ormindale Way
Mississauga, Ontario L5V 1J2
Canada

Jones and Bartlett Publishers
International
Barb House, Barb Mews
London W6 7PA
United Kingdom

Jones and Bartlett's books and products are available through most bookstores and online booksellers. To contact Jones and Bartlett Publishers directly, call 800-832-0034, fax 978-443-8000, or visit our website, www.jbpub.com.

Substantial discounts on bulk quantities of Jones and Bartlett's publications are available to corporations, professional associations, and other qualified organizations. For details and specific discount information, contact the special sales department at Jones and Bartlett via the above contact information or send an email to specialsales@jbpub.com.

The authors, editor, and publisher have made every effort to provide accurate information. However, they are not responsible for errors, omissions, or for any outcomes related to the use of the contents of this book and take no responsibility for the use of the products and procedures described. Treatments and side effects described in this book may not be applicable to all people; likewise, some people may require a dose or experience a side effect that is not described herein. Drugs and medical devices are discussed that may have limited availability controlled by the Food and Drug Administration (FDA) for use only in a research study or clinical trial. Research, clinical practice, and government regulations often change the accepted standard in this field. When consideration is being given to use of any drug in the clinical setting, the healthcare provider or reader is responsible for determining FDA status of the drug, reading the package insert, and reviewing prescribing information for the most up-to-date recommendations on dose, precautions, and contraindications, and determining the appropriate usage for the product. This is especially important in the case of drugs that are new or seldom used.

Production Credits
Acquisitions Editor: Alison Hankey
Editorial Assistant: Sara Cameron
Production Director: Amy Rose
Production Editor: Daniel Stone
V.P., Manufacturing and Inventory Control: Therese Connell
Composition: Auburn Associates, Inc.
Printing and Binding: Malloy, Inc.
Cover Printing: Malloy, Inc.

Cover Credits
Cover Design: Carolyn Downer
Cover Images: Top © Rob Marmion/ShutterStock, Inc.; Bottom Left: © Elena Elisseeva/ShutterStock, Inc.: Bottom Right: © Anna Chelnokova/ShutterStock, Inc.; Inside Front Cover (Author Photo): © David Birnbaum.

Library of Congress Cataloging-in-Publication Data
Chokroverty, Linda.
  100 questions & answers about your child's depression or bipolar disorder / Linda Chokroverty.
    p. cm.
  Includes bibliographical references and index.
  ISBN-13: 978-0-7637-4637-7
  ISBN-10: 0-7637-4637-1
  1. Depression in children—Miscellanea. 2. Manic-depressive illness in children—Miscellanea.
I. Title. II. Title: One hundred questions and answers about your child's depression or bipolar disorder.
  RJ506.D4C475 2010
  618.92'8527—dc22

                                                                                    2009018045

6048

Printed in the United States of America
13 12 11 10 09   10 9 8 7 6 5 4 3 2 1

*This book is dedicated to Maya and Lev,
who made me a better doctor to other children
once I realized the magnitude of parenthood,
and to Craig, my wonderful husband.*

*Special thanks go to all my current and
former patients and their families over the years
who have given me the knowledge to write this book.
Thanks also to my mentors and colleagues who always
have something valuable to teach me, and to my parents
and extended family whose support and guidance have
allowed me to pursue my professional and personal interests.*

Linda Chokroverty, MD, FAAP

Contents

Part 1: Background/The Basics   1

Questions 1–13 describe the basics of depression and bipolar disorder in children, including:

- What types of emotional problems afflict children?
- Do we need to see a psychiatrist to be evaluated and treated for our child's emotional problem? What qualifications does a psychiatrist have to treat children?
- What is a mood disorder? What factors predispose a child to a mood disorder?

Part 2: Risk/Prevention/Epidemiology   25

Questions 14–21 review common causes and reasons behind the emotional disorders, such as:

- How early in childhood is bipolar disorder diagnosed?
- Does depression run in families? What about bipolar disorder?
- What is the prognosis for a child who is diagnosed with a mood disorder?

Part 3: Diagnosis   35

Questions 22–44 discuss how depression and bipolar disorder are diagnosed in children:

- What are the symptoms of depression in a child or adolescent?
- What are the symptoms of bipolar disorder in children?
- What other problems could be associated with a mood disorder?
- How do you manage aggression?

A child's life begins amid great emotion. Their cry announces their arrival into the world. The warm embrace of their parents' joy softens the jolt of birth. And so it goes in the weeks, months, and years to come. Good parents devote much of their time tending to the emotions of their children. So much energy goes into trying to provide the things that make our children happy—play dates, a long sought after gift, or an ice cream cone. A fair amount of toil likewise gets devoted to wiping away tears and allaying anxieties. It is not surprising that so many parents describe how their own happiness is very much contingent upon how their kids are feeling.

When a child's emotions suddenly unfurl beyond the reach of the parent, it is devastating to all. Mood disorders like clinical depression and bipolar disorder leave a child to struggle with severe emotions at a time of life when they are supposed to be developing ways of acknowledging and managing normal emotions. A significant part of human development is devoted to learning how to live a life that is made rich by emotions but not swamped by them. A child with a mood disorder is therefore asked to deal with much more than even most adults can readily handle. Meanwhile you, the parent, are left bereft, helplessly struggling to make it all better as you always could do before. Childhood mood disorders might as well be family mood disorders.

The philosopher Pascal once wrote that "the heart has its reasons, of which reason knows nothing." Our emotional lives, and certainly those of our children, can be confusing and overwhelming. This important book will help you to make some sense of your child's moods, including knowing when you need to turn to a child mental health professional for assistance and understanding the knowledge and ministrations of this professional. The ambitious scope of what follows will help to lend at least some reason to the sometimes turbulent world of your child's emotions.

Craig L. Katz, MD
Clinical Assistant Professor of Psychiatry,
Mount Sinai School of Medicine
Fellow, American Psychiatric Association
President, Disaster Psychiatry Outreach
New York, New York

When I was approached by Jones and Bartlett to write *100 Questions & Answers about Your Child's Depression or Bipolar Disorder*, I had thought at first that it would be too large a topic to cover in a patient education book. Either one of these illnesses (childhood depression or bipolar disorder) would warrant lengthy discussions, and to put them together into a concise book seemed a lofty undertaking. However, as I wrote the book—developing the questions, finding answers, and getting feedback—I was reminded of the continuity at times of the two illnesses, the diagnostic dilemmas experienced by clinicians in distinguishing them, and the different guises that these disorders frequently take over the course of childhood. For a parent without any prior experiences with childhood mental illness, it must be very confusing and intimidating to navigate the sea of information available to the public on these topics. I hope that this book will help make that process a little easier.

This book is aimed at the intelligent reader who is early in the journey to find the best psychiatric care for his or her child. The book assumes a well-established relationship with a primary care doctor such as a pediatrician, and throughout the book, the reader is constantly advised to speak further with the doctor, whether it is a pediatrician or a psychiatrist. I would seek pardon from the majority of mental health professionals, my colleagues who are not physicians but who provide the lion's share of care to children suffering from mood disorders, for my frequent references to "your doctor" in the book. Being a doctor, I have been trained to think of the doctor as a major force behind treatment, but I recognize that taking care of children, mentally healthy or otherwise, requires the input from a number of adult professionals, ranging from educators to therapists with a variety of backgrounds, not to mention responsible parents. On the other hand, much of what I refer the reader to inquire about with their doctor is often related to specific matters of diagnosis, medications, and physiology, which is certainly the doctor's area of expertise.

After having worked with so many parents to help clarify the nature of their child's illness, and having taught child psychiatry trainees for a number of years about the basic elements of psychiatric diagnosis, I find that the opportunity to write this book has come at a rather good time. I thank the team at Jones and Bartlett for their patience and perseverance in preparing this book. I am grateful for the chance to help even more families through this book grapple the issues that they are being asked to face with an ill child. I am constantly humbled as my own children grow, with the trials and tribulations of basic parenting, to think about the tremendous stress and challenges faced by parents who must try to go above and beyond what I must do.

Linda Chokroverty, MD, FAAP

Geraldine Harris and her husband, Steve, are the parents of a son and daughter, both of whom have emotional disturbances. Their son, Joseph (11), is the more stable of the two children at this time, experiencing symptoms of inattention and low mood that fall below the levels that are considered diagnosable. Nonetheless, he receives additional educational services in school to help with his impairments. Their daughter, Lexie (10), continues to undergo assessments and treatment for her diagnosis of a depressive disorder and attention deficit hyperactivity disorder (ADHD). Lexie and her family have been struggling with her behaviors since she was a preschooler. The family has sought services from a number of mental health and educational professionals in the community. In addition to her treatments for ADHD, Lexie is about to start antidepressant medication for her symptoms of depression.

The Harris family lives about an hour from Philadelphia and both children attend their local public school. Geraldine is a sociology professor at a local college and her husband has his own business in computer programming.

PART ONE

Background/ The Basics

What types of emotional problems afflict children?

Do we need to see a psychiatrist to be evaluated and treated for our child's emotional problem? What qualifications does a psychiatrist have to treat children?

What is a mood disorder? What factors predispose a child to a mood disorder?

More . . .

1. What are the different areas of growth and development that a child undergoes in becoming an adult? How is development related to emotional problems in children?

From the time we first hold our precious child in our arms, we are immediately struck by the fact that she will grow in all dimensions. The various dimensions of growth include physical, motor, cognitive, social, and emotional development.

The first area of growth that is apparent to us in our child is *physical growth*. A baby is tiny and helpless at first, but quickly you watch her become bigger, more mobile and independent. Her body changes from having a large head, a chubby face, hands and feet, to that of a little girl, later an awkward preteen, then eventually she becomes a young adult who may even resemble you.

Accompanying physical growth is *motor development*—learning to sit, walk, run, balance, dance, and other actions. More complicated motor skills that require combination with thinking and learning (see the next paragraph) include the ability to draw and write, play sports or instruments, and so on.

Another significant area of growth in a child is centered in the brain's ability to think, learn, and have memory, referred to as *cognitive development*. Even as an infant, this development is obvious as she learns how a toy works or how to play make-believe. What we think of as the more sophisticated brain functions falls under the category of cognitive development—

problem solving, academic activities, etc. A child's achievement throughout school and acquiring knowledge is an example of cognitive development. The complicated task of speaking, in one or more languages, requires both thinking and motor skills (of the mouth) to be highly developed.

An area of growth that is less obvious at first, but soon proves to be as important as the others, is *social development*. An infant first shows this by interacting with his mother, responding and taking in cues from the environment about how to smile, greet people, laugh, and enjoy the company of other babies. Later, he will learn to make friends, share toys, and play games with other children. As an older child and teenager, he will want the approval of his peers, share in common interests and hobbies, or perhaps engage in competition with others. Throughout his childhood and adolescence, he will learn about the appropriateness and context of his words and actions as they impact on other people. He will develop ways of resolving conflicts, whether it is how to share a toy with a sibling, negotiate his first summer job, or handle challenges when he is a father of young children himself.

Emotional development is especially complex and integrates all of the other aspects of development already mentioned, plus the ability to regulate one's feelings using cues from the outside world. A baby intuitively has feelings of happiness, frustration, and irritability. He learns to seek validation or comfort from his mother and those who love him when these feelings arise. Eventually he will be able to soothe himself without the adults, at least for minor challenges to his frustration. As a toddler, he has difficulty controlling his impulses and his anger, often throwing tantrums

Emotional development is especially complex and integrates all of the other aspects of development already mentioned, plus the ability to regulate one's feelings using cues from the outside world.

and showing aggression, but gradually learns otherwise from his parents and nurturing adults who help him by setting the right examples, setting limits, and letting him know he is still loved. He starts to realize that he can control his own body and what it does. Later, as a preschooler and school-aged child, he will be better able to show restraint, master his temper and voice tone, and use words rather than actions to communicate his wishes. Confidence and self-esteem evolve further in the school-aged child. In high school, a teenager becomes exquisitely aware of his feelings and starts to appreciate relationships he has with his family members and other people in the world. Even into his 20s, a young adult is still developing in this domain and many would argue that full emotional maturity is not reached until at least this stage, if not later.

While we see our child growing up, outward changes along these dimensions correspond to internal growth and maturation of all the organs and systems within the body, on both a macroscopic and the microscopic level. In this book, we will focus on the developing nervous system which is comprised of the brain and nerves. Unlike other parts of the body, the brain is equipped at birth with almost all the cells it will need in a lifetime. However, these cells are immature and underdeveloped in the early years and the tasks of the brain in these first years of infancy and childhood are to increase and refine the numbers of connections between these cells and to allow production of an important substance known as myelin. Like a tree extending its branches in a forest of other such trees, the microscopic "branches" of the brain, extensions of the nerve cells, develop millions of connections to and from each other and in between, and serve as the means of communication for the body. On the smallest scale, each nerve cell's connection to the next facilitates not only an important function like seeing, moving, feeling, etc., but also can represent a new learning experience. Another process equally important as the formation of all these connections is the process of trimming back or "pruning" of all the nerve branches in the brain throughout childhood and adolescence. This process is similar to the need to prune the excess foliage on a rose bush to allow for the best flowers to grow. Still using the tree metaphor, just as a sapling forms bark to better strengthen itself and preserve the contents within, many cells of the brain and nerves of an infant and young child produce a special material, myelin, which helps support the growth of cells and improve the speed and efficiency of the transportation. Thus, two major areas of growth in a child's brain and nervous system correspond to the increases and decreases in the different connections, and the laying down of myelin.

Developmental theorists try to explain the causes of emotional disturbance in children. Some feel the disturbance reflects a change in the normal course of development due to factors related to the environment or biological tendencies within the child. Others believe a child's lack of age-appropriate skills to navigate development is a root cause of emotional disturbance. There are those who believe that a failure to progress from one stage of development to the next has occurred in the case of certain emotional and behavioral disorders. For example, the hyperactivity seen in toddlers is generally considered normal at that age, but when persistent after kindergarten or first grade, it becomes disruptive and problematic in school and other environments and may be classified as attention deficit hyperactivity disorder (ADHD). In the toddler and preschool years, a child may become irritable for a variety of reasons, but as various skills to cope with frustration are learned, the duration and intensity of such irritability typically diminishes as he gets older. For a variety of reasons that include intrinsic factors of the child such as biology, as well as extrinsic factors such as environment and life experiences, a child with depression or bipolar disorder can be very irritable at times. The irritability of such a child may illustrate a developmental crisis where skills to counteract frustration were inadequately formed. Some of these children may have presented with this kind of irritability or difficulty managing frustration from a very young age, and only later in childhood or adolescence, present with the constellation of symptoms of a mood disorder.

It is also important for parents to appreciate the role of development in their child's emotional problem because it will guide the types of treatment that may be appropriate.

The reason to mention development in the context of mental illness in a child or adolescent is rather obvious; the child is constantly changing and growing despite being afflicted with an illness, and both growth and illness will affect the progress of the other. It is also important for parents to appreciate the role of development in their child's emotional problem because it will guide the types of treatment that may be appropriate. As children with emotional disorders grow up, they may be fortunate to learn how to manage problems more effectively as part of their treatment as well as the maturational process. This is often achieved through the combined efforts of families and their doctors. It helps parents see their child and her behavior more as a work in progress, rather than a single problem that must be "fixed."

2. When can a child communicate her feelings effectively? Why won't my child tell me what's wrong with her?

It's not uncommon for a child, especially a preschooler, to say "I don't know," when her mother asks her what's wrong. It's usually not because your daughter is trying to be defiant or difficult by answering this way, but rather because the ability to interpret one's own feelings and then express them back to someone else requires a high level of sophistication that she may not yet have achieved. Not only are the demands of the proper use of language and vocabulary needed, but also the social context and cues, a child's individual style, the family's use of language, and many other factors necessary to convey information using spoken words. Once your daughter has a basic command of spoken language—in the preschool years, for example, she can let you know how she feels in a rudimentary way— "I'm happy, I'm sad....". It may take her many years, however, to be effective at understanding and communicating subtle and complicated feelings. This is why adolescents may feel "confused"; they are overwhelmed with so many experiences and ideas that they just don't know how to sort it all out in a coherent way to others, especially adults. (Adolescents also have another active period of brain maturation that may further add to the experience of being overwhelmed at times by different feelings.)

Don't take it too hard if your daughter is not telling you what you want to hear about feelings. Every child is different in his rate of being able to communicate well. Some are able to do it earlier, others later, and some have a difficult time doing it throughout life. In many ways we, as adults, spend our whole lifetime learning to be more effective at communicating about our feelings to others. Problems in marriage and social relationships such as those with coworkers are common among adults who continue to struggle with communication. Knowing this, we must constantly remind ourselves that our children, like us, are "in process" and that we need to be patient and find ways of bringing out what we want from them. Various treatments for emotional problems focus on identifying feelings, finding ways of expressing them, and managing them. Many cultures don't talk about feelings at all, so it becomes an added challenge to learn to do this if your family is not accustomed to verbalizing internal experiences. Your doctor may provide a wealth of information about how a child develops the important skill of communication, and you should feel free to ask more about it.

Geraldine's comment:

The issue of communication on the part of a child is interesting. Recently, my daughter who is 10 years old asked, "What's ADHD?" It was the first time after all these years of evaluations, treatments, etc., that it was even given a name. The grownups had not addressed this at all with her in these terms, but instead it was about describing the behaviors. It made me realize that she was capable of having a conversation about some of the things we'd all been struggling with up until now.

On the matter of other professionals like teachers and so forth picking up on problems, it was the daycare that first thought Lexie needed services at the age of 3. She had more trouble initiating activities, during transitions, etc., compared to other children. She was referred for evaluation by a preschool committee on special education. She then received special services at first in the home. A social worker would visit us once a month and work with her on socialization skills, game playing, etc. She assessed her, and provided us with family support. Because we were educated professionals, the therapist presumed that we knew more than we really knew, which was not a good thing. I think therapists need to be as objective as they can in their work, and make no assumptions about the families.

3. Why does my child need help emotionally? There's nothing wrong with her!

Acknowledging that your child has an emotional problem is very hard. After all, what parent wants to admit that their child is not keeping up with other children in the area of emotional development? It may be easier not to deal with the problem than to admit that something is wrong. Some parents may accept that a child's behavior (which is often the outward expression of the child's emotional state), whether appropriate or not, is just "the way it is" and that this feature is part of the child's personality and cannot or should not be changed. Many parents are able to characterize their children and accept that "he is a cranky boy," or "she is a shy girl," or even that "she is a sad girl." A mother or father who has known the child for so many years may have gotten used to how he behaves, unless of course, other people in the child's life, such as a teacher, or other relatives express concern about how the child is functioning or appearing to them. At times, it may be hard to tease apart what traits are part of a child's constitution, what traits have arisen anew, and which ones warrant treatment. However, as a general rule, if your child is having trouble in school or at home with siblings or other family members

. . . as a general rule, if your child is having trouble in school or at home with siblings or other family members in a way that he is just not functioning well, it is a good idea to seek further guidance.

in a way that he is just not functioning well, it is a good idea to seek further guidance. Teachers and pediatricians are important professionals with whom your child has a relationship and who may be able offer such guidance. Teachers are very well informed about the social and academic functioning of a child in their class. They often have considerable experience with children and may identify those who need help. Your child's teacher may have already recognized that your child is not doing well and recommended help. In such a case, your child or your family may be referred to a counselor in school who can spend more time on the situation and help you understand if professional help is advised. The other important professional who may be able to offer guidance to the family about a child who is functioning poorly in the community is your pediatrician. Pediatricians are highly familiar with normal childhood development and are resources for parents who need help recognizing when a child appears to fall outside the range of normal in the area of emotional development. Once a professional such as a teacher or pediatrician has recommended more help, it crucial that you take this suggestion seriously.

Perhaps you are a parent who has sensed all along that something is different about your child's behavior or disposition, and you've wondered if you should seek help, but have been hesitant to do so. Be aware that "help" may mean only further clarification on whether a child's behaviors or emotional experiences are "normal," or it could also mean referral to a mental health professional for evaluation and treatment of a more serious emotional disorder.

Once a problem is identified, your child's well-being and future depend on your ability as a parent to get help as soon as you can.

Once a problem is identified, your child's well-being and future depend on your ability as a parent to get help as soon as you can. As with any other childhood medical problem, like an infection or an injury, an emotional problem needs to be addressed right away to help your child recover and achieve optimal growth and development.

4. What types of emotional problems afflict children?

In some regards, children and adolescents experience similar emotional illnesses as adults. Examples of these include depression, anxiety, bipolar disorder, schizophrenia, substance abuse problems, sleep disorders, and a number of other disorders. But, people who work with children professionally will usually tell you "children are not little adults." What they mean is that the presentation of childhood illnesses appear very differently, and can therefore be more challenging to identify and treat. Some emotional and/or behavioral disorders present almost exclusively in childhood, but often persist into adulthood, at times in a different guise or to a lesser extent. These include autism and related developmental disorders, attention deficit hyperactivity disorder (ADHD) and other disruptive behavioral disorders, learning disorders, communication disorders, mental retardation, problems with feeding and elimination, neurologic disorders known as tics, and certain problems with relatedness to important caregivers known as attachment disorders.

In this book, only the **mood disorders**, previously known as affective disorders, will be discussed. These include major depressive disorder (MDD), other variations of depression, and the different types of bipolar disorder (BPD).

Mood Disorders

Any of several types of depression or bipolar disorders that are defined in the Diagnostic and Statistical Manual (DSM).

Biogenic amines

Three neurotransmitters traditionally associated with mood and anxiety disorders. These include dopamine, norepinephrine, and serotonin.

Dopamine

Neurotransmitter associated with pleasure seeking and reward, motor functions in the body (movement), attention and organizational skills.

Norepinephrine

A neurotransmitter involved with attention, associated with the "fight or flight" response that acts upon heart rate and blood pressure, and is involved with arousal and wakefulness.

Serotonin

A neurotransmitter associated with control of mood, appetite, memory, and sleep.

5. What are neurotransmitters? How do they control how we feel?

Neurotransmitters are chemicals that exist within the body, which transport different kinds of information along the cells of the brain and nervous system. The transport occurs through chemical reactions, electrical activity, or both. Neurotransmitters are among hundreds of different chemicals that influence the body. They come in different sizes, some very small and simple in their chemical structure, and others quite large and complex. The activity of neurotransmitters and other chemicals also varies from simple to complex, involving a few or many events. The movement and activity of an important group of neurotransmitters, known as the **biogenic amines**, are responsible for emotions, thinking, and behavior. The biogenic amines consist of three important neurotransmitters implicated in a variety of psychiatric disorders. These three are **dopamine, norepinephrine**, and **serotonin**. Each of these neurotransmitters has characteristic functions in the nervous system. For example, the neurotransmitter dopamine is involved with attention, motivation, feeling pleasure and reward, and other experiences such as hallucinations.

Problems with the activity of dopamine can result in psychiatric disorders as varied as ADHD, cocaine abuse, or schizophrenia. Medications used to treat psychiatric disorders affect dopamine and the other neurotransmitters, serotonin and norepinephrine. You'll read more about these specific neurotransmitters, especially serotonin, when medications are discussed later in the section on treatment.

6. Do we need to see a psychiatrist to be evaluated and treated for our child's emotional problem? What qualifications does a psychiatrist have to treat children?

The most likely person to be made aware of a child's emotional problem by a parent is the primary care doctor, usually a pediatrician or family doctor. The problems might be discussed during a visit for general health care. Parents often have an intimate and long-standing relationship with their child's pediatrician, since they have known this doctor ever since their child was a baby, and may feel most comfortable bringing such problems to her attention. Some pediatricians have the additional skills, time, and comfort level to treat certain emotional problems such as attention deficit hyperactivity disorder (ADHD) and depression in children. Given her busy schedule in the practice, the type of treatment a pediatrician can offer for these problems is usually in the form of medication and possibly some emotional support. Beyond this, many pediatricians do not feel they have the training to treat more complicated emotional problems, since their expertise is usually in physical medicine. They may choose to refer the child to a social worker in their own practice if available, a mental health clinic, or to a private psychologist or psychiatrist for further evaluation and more comprehensive treatment.

If seeing a psychiatrist is recommended, that may stir up a lot of feelings in parents. In our society, the idea of a psychiatrist brings various images to mind. Literature, the media, and history have all contributed to these notions. Some of these are humorous and rather

Background / The Basics

fantastic, and others are quite negative and troubling. When many people think of a psychiatrist, it still invokes an image of Freud conducting "analysis" on a vulnerable, reclining individual. Having to see a psychiatrist may invoke fears and insecurities of being scrutinized, "diagnosed" with terrible problems, or simply being labeled as "crazy." People still have assumptions about the treatments offered by a psychiatrist, which may involve being locked up on a hospital ward, put in a strait jacket, kept among raving lunatics, or even being subjected to electrocution and removal of parts of the brain. Society can also be judgmental of a person who seeks the help of a psychiatrist due to distortions of who the psychiatrist is, and what diagnosis or treatment from a psychiatrist implies about the individual. I once saw a child at the urgency of a school guidance counselor who correctly realized that the child was in need of psychiatric help. However, efforts to engage the parents revealed that the family was humiliated by the idea of interacting with a psychiatrist and, sadly, the child continued to suffer. For the sake of that child and others in the future, it's imperative to debunk the myth of the psychiatrist.

A psychiatrist is a medical doctor who has had extensive education and training in the field of human emotions and behavior, and treatment of its problems.

A psychiatrist is a medical doctor who has had extensive education and training in the field of human emotions and behavior, and treatment of its problems. The psychiatrist graduated from college and medical school, is licensed to practice medicine in whatever state she lives in, and has additional training in the practice of general psychiatry. If the doctor is a child psychiatrist, she has further specialty training in normal and abnormal child development, diagnosis and treatment of emotional problems in children and adolescents. Once all the education and training has been completed, she is eligible to take one or more examinations in psychiatry, known as the "boards" and, once she successfully completes these examinations, she is "board-certified" in the field of general psychiatry, and possibly other subspecialized fields such as child psychiatry. While a license is required for all practicing physicians, only a percentage of them will also be board-certified, which is a measure of professional distinction and qualification, but not a requirement. In addition, psychiatrists may be further trained in various types of treatments, such as certain psychotherapies, which require additional training. To complement all this intellectual training, a psychiatrist will have acquired practical experience in treating patients ranging anywhere from a few years to decades. A psychiatrist maintains the same standards as all other physicians with regard to confidentiality and record keeping. Depending on her interests, she may treat children with any number of non-pharmacologic (not involving medicines) methods such as psychotherapy and/or with medications. Some psychiatrists provide only medical evaluation, medications, and monitoring as treatment. In these cases, another clinician such as a therapist with a background in mental health (e.g., a social worker or psychologist) sees a child more frequently and the psychiatrist sees him periodically for medications, but both communicate with each other and work together toward common treatment goals for the child.

If you have a choice between a general psychiatrist and a child psychiatrist, it will be helpful to choose the latter, as she will have more training and experience specifically with children. However, the United States has a shortage of child psychiatrists and if you live in an area that is remote or underserved by specialized doctors, you may not have a choice. If you must seek

If you have a choice between a general psychiatrist and a child psychiatrist, it will be helpful to choose the latter, as she will have more training and experience specifically with children.

15

out the services of a general psychiatrist, ask her what experience she has in treating children and adolescents and try to find the most experienced one available.

7. What other professionals are qualified to treat emotional disorders in children?

In addition to psychiatrists, other professionals treat children's emotional problems. In fact, the majority of people who treat children for emotional problems are not psychiatrists at all, but rather social workers, psychologists, psychiatric nurse practitioners, art therapists, substance abuse counselors, family therapists, and various other counselors with backgrounds in child therapy. This group is often referred to as "mental health professionals" or "therapists." Any of these clinicians may engage children and families in psychotherapy ("talk therapy") or other nonverbal treatments such as play, music, drama, dance, etc. Some are highly trained and have earned advanced degrees, and others are less trained. Psychologists are often trained to perform diagnostic testing in addition to highly organized types of therapy. In the United States, only certain professionals are permitted to prescribe medications. These professionals include licensed physicians, but in certain parts of the country, also nurse practitioners, physician's assistants, and in one state, licensed psychologists with training in psychiatric medications.

Schools, particularly high schools, may have a mental health professional on staff as part of their guidance department as well. Some educational professionals with additional training in therapy also treat children. Many school guidance counselors will see children for "counseling" in mental health issues, but usually will not evaluate and treat them in the same depth as a trained mental health professional. They can, however, be very encouraging and supportive of the child and family, and may recommend further assessment by a qualified expert. In any case, always seek out a professional who is reputable in the community, and has experience in treating children.

In some parts of the United States, and much of the world, a pediatrician or other primary care doctor is the only one available to treat a child's emotional problems. Some of these physicians are comfortable with this, but a large percentage of them are not. In such cases further consultation, by phone, teleconference or special training sessions with the necessary mental health professionals such as psychiatrists may be sought to better serve such children.

Geraldine's comment:
I would add developmental-behavioral pediatricians and pediatric neurologists also to this list of other professionals certainly qualified to evaluate children with emotional problems, and possibly treat them, too. One of the most helpful assessments Lexie got for school was done by a developmental-behavioral pediatrician. I would highly recommend this person to other families. We are currently seeing a pediatric neurologist for our daughter.

8. What causes depression? Did we cause our son's depression by being strict or using severe punishment? Did we cause it by getting a divorce? Can a death in the family cause childhood depression?

Current thinking in the field suggests that there is no single cause of depression in a child. Rather, the coincidence of many factors is believed to influence whether a child becomes depressed or has another mental illness. An inherited, chemical predisposition to depression, a poor relationship between the parent and child, a depressed parent, life stressors such as major illness, loss of important loved ones, being a victim or witness to violence, or sexual abuse are just a few possible risk factors for depression. Usually, one event or risk factor does not cause it, and can be tolerated by the child. More likely, a number of events and personal risk factors have added up over time and contributed to your son's depression. As a parent, it can be hard to think that something you did or that happened in your son's upbringing has caused him to be depressed. Sometimes, there is no simple answer to explain the depression. If knowing how or why this happened is important to you, exploring this issue in your son's treatment is a good idea.

At times, we have little control over the events or personal risk factors that contribute to the development of depression in our children. In other cases, such as those where parental depression and other emotional problems are undertreated (see also Question 91), there may be circumstances in which a child's mental health is strongly influenced by the parent. In these cases, an opportunity exists for the parents to regain some control over the situation and modify the risk factors for their child's depression by getting help for their own problems. For many families, understanding the causes of their child's depression can help lessen the guilt experienced, and may help in the recovery process as well.

For many families, understanding the causes of their child's depression can help lessen the guilt experienced, and may help in the recovery process as well.

9. Why do some children experience emotional problems, whereas others who endure the same kinds of stress do not?

This ties into the last question and answer about the additive nature of emotional problems. Often, a child will be "hit" by a number of different stressors, and her "system" will be unable to handle it all, the end result being mental illness (the multi-hit hypothesis). Also, some children are better able to withstand different life stressors and have more adaptive abilities than others. This feature in such children is known as **resilience.** Children who still manage to have a better attitude and successful life despite the odds are considered to be more resilient than other children with a similar experience, who did not do as well. This is commonly seen among siblings of a child with depression, who may not experience the disabling illness even though they have been raised in a similar way with similar genetic influences. Resilience is felt to be a special characteristic that is part of a child's constitution.

Resilience

The ability for some children to adapt or succeed despite adversity.

10. What is a mood disorder? What factors predispose a child to a mood disorder?

The *Diagnostic and Statistical Manual of Mental Disorders, 4th Edition* (*DSM*) categorizes illnesses that are characterized by depression, mania, or both as mood disorders. (In psychiatry, "mood" refers to the subjective way a person feels inside—e.g., sad, happy, anxious, etc.). Depression is a term that describes a prolonged period of sad or irritable mood, along with other symptoms. Mania is another mood state, characterized by a prolonged period of elevated or irritable mood, also with other symptoms. Mood disorders can arise independently, or can be the result of a medical illness or substance abuse problem. (More specific descriptions of depression and mania are given in Part 3: Diagnosis.) In children and adolescents, the biggest risk factor associated with a mood disorder is having an immediate relative (a "first-degree relative" such as a sibling or a parent) with a mood disorder. Children with a parent who has other psychiatric problems such as substance abuse are also at risk. The reasons for this are felt to be both biological (genetically inherited brain structure or chemistry from the parent) and psychosocial or environmental (problematic parent-child relationships or a chaotic home life that arise from having an impaired parent). Other risks for developing a mood disorder include a child having another psychiatric disorder earlier in childhood, such as ADHD, or an anxiety disorder. Female gender seems to predispose a child toward depression, because adolescent girls have a higher risk for depression than boys (see also Question 16). Environmental risks include having a family environment with a number of conflicts (frequent arguments between the parents, between parents and children, or among siblings, domestic violence) or poor communication style within the family. Other risks include the inability for a child to handle overwhelming stressors of life such as life-threatening situations, abuse, or profound losses such as the death of a parent.

11. What factors are protective against mood disorder?

Several factors are considered protective for children against psychiatric disorders in general, including the mood disorders. These include individual characteristics of the child, as well as family or environmental traits. On the individual level, a child who is easy to get along with, adapts to change without too much difficulty, communicates well with others, has interests that occupy her, can soothe herself when distressed, is intelligent, and independent, displays some of the features that protect against emotional disorders. Family traits that are protective include having a solid relationship with an important caregiver such as a parent, and the availability of other adults such as grandparents or extended family members to help in raising the child and emotionally support the parent. Factors within the environment or community that are protective include connection with a supportive religious group such as a church, parental employment and financial stability, enrollment in a school that is safe and nurturing, and a connection with a supportive teacher or other positive adult role models.

12. Why talk about depression and bipolar disorder in the same discussion? Aren't they two different illnesses?

Major depressive disorder (MDD), a special type of depression, and bipolar disorder (BPD), are classified in the DSM as separate disorders with different characteristics. However, they are often related and, as mentioned previously, fall under the general category of mood disorders. Experience with youth suffering from BPD shows that they frequently present with depression when they first become ill. In those youngsters, other symptoms unique to BPD, such as mania, present at a later time which then clarify the diagnosis. Furthermore, many people with BPD have depression as part of their pattern of illness. Often the depression and bipolar symptoms go hand in hand.

The common symptoms are not the only reason to consider the two illnesses together. The treatments for the disorders, particularly from a medication standpoint, can be similar, although those with BPD will probably have a slightly more complicated regimen. If medications are indicated for depression, an antidepressant may be used. Pharmacologic treatment of BPD may also include an antidepressant, but certain precautions and considerations are made in these cases. More about treatment will be mentioned in later questions.

The relationship between the two disorders is intriguing and is usually a relevant topic of discussion in your child's therapy.

13. What are the consequences of untreated mood disorders in children?

Some parents are unaware of the need to treat, or are against the treatment of, their child's mood disorders, and may choose to "let it be" and hope that things will resolve on their own. However, leaving well enough alone is not always a good thing. A child who is sad or irritable all the time may not be able to keep up in school because she is not able to focus on the work. She may become further discouraged and miss school chronically, which can lead to academic delays, social isolation, and poor social development. Some children may never finish school and compromise their future as productive adults. Teenagers with untreated mood disorders can take greater risks such as engaging in unprotected sex or drug use, and put themselves in dangerous situations with other risk-taking youths. Some adolescent girls may become pregnant for the wrong reasons. In an effort to numb or forget the overwhelming feelings experienced, a teenager with a mood disorder might smoke, drink, or abuse illegal substances, and become dependent on them. He could engage in criminal activities to support his drug habits. School dropout, pregnancy, drugs, and crime are just a few of the consequences of untreated mood disorders.

Every so often, we hear about very sad events, where troubled young people turn violence on their own communities, taking innocent lives. These individuals often needed help for mood disorders and other complicated social problems they may have had. Aggression, toward others or even oneself, in the form of suicide, is the ultimate and devastating end result of untreated depression or BPD. In all, so many more risks are taken by *not* treating a child's mood disorder

Some parents are unaware of the need to treat, or are against the treatment of, their child's mood disorders, and may choose to "let it be" and hope that things will resolve on their own.

that it is compels a parent to seek help right away when a problem is apparent, before it can lead to any number of tragic outcomes.

Geraldine's comment:

I worry a lot for Lexie's future. I worry that she might be pushed into premature sex and other activities, as she is overly curious at times, and doesn't always use good discretion. I worry that I will have to be around for her for life.

PART TWO

Risk, Prevention, and Epidemiology

How early in childhood is bipolar disorder diagnosed?

Does depression run in families? What about bipolar disorder?

What is the prognosis for a child who is diagnosed with a mood disorder?

More . . .

14. How often do mood disorders strike children?

Depressive disorders and bipolar disorders occur at different rates. Depressive disorders are seen at a rate of about 2% of children, and between 4–8% of adolescents. Bipolar disorders occur far less frequently than depressive disorders. Bipolar disorder occurs at a rate of about 1% in older adolescents and young adults. It has long been assumed that young children are rarely diagnosed with it. Studies of adults with bipolar disorder, looking back on their childhood, show that far below the 1% were stricken with the illness before they were 10 years old. Yet, other studies reveal that adults with bipolar disorder suffered symptoms for many years before their illness became known. The phenomenon of "juvenile bipolar disorder" has become a hot topic for debate in recent years in the field of child psychiatry. Some experts in the field now suggest that the rate in children could be close to that of adults, due to the observation that the first presentation of bipolar disorder in children is frequently one of depression, with mania presenting as a symptom in a later episode of illness. Also, many doctors are seeing symptoms of bipolar disorder in children that may not fulfill all the criteria of a traditional diagnosis, but nonetheless fall on the spectrum of the illness, and may benefit from the treatments for the disorder. Finally, professionals are often faced with diagnostic challenges, since some of the symptoms of BPD, such as hyperactivity and impulsivity, are common in other disorders such as ADHD, and could be mistaken for the other disorder. Adding further to this diagnostic dilemma is the fact that studies suggest that ADHD and BPD often occur together in children, and may pose further delay in diagnosis and treatment of the BPD. Thus, for a variety of reasons, young adults and teens who receive a diagnosis BPD at a later age may have had it earlier in their life, but it was not recognized as bipolar disorder.

15. Do girls get depression more often than boys?

In earlier childhood, girls and boys have equal rates of depression in most cultures. In the United States and other industrialized cultures, by adolescence—above age 12, girls become depressed twice as often as boys. Why this happens is not fully understood, but may be related to various factors. Some of the reasons may include the change in hormone levels associated with puberty, or the appearance of puberty at an earlier age in girls than boys and the consequences associated with this event. Psychosocial issues, such as societal roles for girls that are more restrictive than those for boys, increased risk of sexual abuse in girls, the tendency for girls to be more reflective, and girls having more concerns about body image may also explain their higher rate of depression in adolescence.

16. How early in childhood is bipolar disorder diagnosed?

Bipolar disorder (BPD) is an illness that is generally diagnosed in the late teens to early adulthood. The Epidemiologic Catchment Area study reported that the mean age of onset for BPD was 21, with the most cases arising between the ages of 15–19. Traditionally, it was considered rare in childhood, and occasional in early adolescence. However, looking back at their childhoods, adult patients with bipolar disorder can

Bipolar disorder (BPD) is an illness that is generally diagnosed in the late teens to early adulthood.

27

describe symptoms of the illness that occurred when they were children but might not have been picked up or treated. The literature on BPD has revealed that often the diagnosis is not made until many years—as many as 10—following the onset of symptoms. The disorder is being studied more and more, and the definitions of BPD ("bipolarity") have been expanded in recent times. For example, symptoms of the illness such as hypomania or frequent, shorter bouts of manic behavior, known as **cyclothymia**, are seen more often in children and adolescents over the classic manic episodes observed in adults. As a result, increasing numbers of children are being diagnosed and treated by child psychiatrists at a younger age than in the past. Experts on BPD, such as Dr. Barbara Geller at Washington University and others, have even observed that the illness takes on different characteristics when it occurs in the younger teen or preteen years. Those children who are diagnosed with the disorder at the youngest ages tend to have more severe symptoms, a more chronic, even continuous course of illness (as opposed to episodic), and are usually male. While BPD will occasionally be diagnosed in a child, it is rare that a child psychiatrist will diagnose a toddler or preschooler with bipolar disorder, since a child's developmental stage (e.g., communication skills, emotional regulation, relationship with parents and environment) at these ages makes it difficult, if not impossible, to apply typical diagnostic criteria (derived primarily from adult studies). However, there are experts in the field who specialize in such young children who may be able to help understand whether a child fits into the early stages of a mood disorder. Adding to the confusion, studies have shown that people with BPD often present with depression before mania. This situation may lead doctors and families to believe that the child

Cyclothymia

Also referred to as "cyclothymic disorder." According to the *DSM*, in children and adolescents cyclothymic disorder is diagnosed when a year or more of numerous periods of hypomanic and depressive symptoms, along with other criteria are observed (see Table 6). It is used in cases where BPD or MDD is difficult to determine because the fluctuations of mood are often too rapid, too short in duration, or too mild in severity to fit the usual definition of these disorders.

has a depressive disorder, which will only later be confirmed as bipolar illness.

Like the phenomenon of ADHD, BPD in children is being diagnosed more frequently than in the past, especially among those being seen in private doctors' offices. Some professionals may feel it is being over-diagnosed, whereas others may feel it's often missed. Your doctor may be able to discuss this topic with you in further detail as it is a complicated one that has been a matter of controversy and confusion in recent years, even among professionals.

17. At what age is depression usually diagnosed in children?

By the time a youngster reaches adulthood, about one in five will have experienced major depression. Most of these cases of depression will occur in the teenage years ("post-pubertal age"). Children have been described by researchers and clinicians to have depression as young as 3 years of age; even babies and toddlers, using a specialized set of criteria that are modifications of the those in the *DSM* (The Zero to Three Criteria), have been observed to have depression. Therefore, the short answer to this question is that most cases of depression are diagnosed after age 12, but can, on occasion, occur earlier.

By the time a youngster reaches adulthood, about one in five will have experienced major depression.

18. Does depression run in families? What about bipolar disorder?

Both depression and BPD can be inherited, and having an immediate relative such as a parent or a sibling (a first degree relative) with the disorder puts the child at much higher risk than the general population to develop it. Children with a depressed parent are 3–10 times more likely to have depression, and those with a parent with BPD are up to 6–10 times more likely to have bipolar illness. However, the transmission of a mood disorder is not due only to the genes between parents and children. Having an ill parent can confer a biologically inherited, as well as an environmentally created risk for the child.

19. What is the prognosis for a child who is diagnosed with a mood disorder?

Prognosis for mood disorders and a variety of other emotional problems is based on a number of conditions.

Prognosis for mood disorders and a variety of other emotional problems is based on a number of conditions. For example, when depression or BPD strikes at a younger age—such as before puberty, the prognosis is more guarded than when it occurs in an older age. With BPD in particular, a younger child with the diagnosis may have a more severe presentation than an older one, and experience more psychosocial disability in the form of poor relationships with family members, disturbance in the classroom that might cause academic delays, and more accumulation of negative life experiences related to symptoms of the illness. Important aspects of normal psychosocial development are frequently interfered with during mood disorder episodes, and this can have a dramatic effect on a younger child. With the exception of ADHD, younger children with psychiatric disturbances frequently have a lower response rate to psychotropic medications as compared to adults, and may suffer longer. The reasons for this poorer response rate may include environmental stressors that may continue to exist despite the treatment, and the fact that children may be metabolizing psychiatric medications differently than adults.

Other conditions that could further complicate treatment, recovery, and ultimately the prognosis of a mood disorder include the presence of other illnesses (termed **comorbid conditions** in psychiatry) such as ADHD, behaviors that cause problems with the law, or learning difficulties. Concurrent drug or alcohol abuses with mood disorders are associated with a worse prognosis as well.

Comorbid conditions

The presence of two or more psychiatric disorders in the same individual. An example would be having ADHD and depression.

Some conditions within the child and family can make for a better prognosis, while others make for a worse one. Better prognosis is associated with having a caring and intact family, and having a supportive extended community for the child and parents. More guarded prognosis is observed among children who have emotionally troubled parents who are not in treatment, have excessively stressful life circumstances, and those who have experienced sexual abuse.

A careful assessment of your child's situation and treatment options will help you and your doctor anticipate prognosis for the future.

20. What are the chances that my daughter will have another manic episode once she has been diagnosed?

A sobering fact is that mood disorders generally have a recurring pattern to the illness, despite all the advances in treatment. It is unusual for a single episode of mania or depression to be followed by lifelong recovery from the symptoms. According to the American Psychiatric

Association (APA), adults with untreated BPD may have more than 10 episodes of mania and depression in a lifetime. Research with children and adolescents with BPD also shows that, as with adults, recurrences of such episodes are frequent. Dr. Boris Birmaher at the University of Pittsburgh and his colleagues interviewed more than 260 children and adolescents who had BPD from clinics and hospitals and found that half of them had one or more recurrences in a 2-year period, often depressive episodes. They also found that a high percentage of these patients, about 70% of them, recovered fully from the first episode of either mania or depression. Some years earlier, Dr. Maria Kovacs conducted a literature review on the course of depression, and noted that children and adolescents recovered from their first depressive episodes faster than adults, but had a 60% chance of recurrence. These figures and others suggest that your daughter has an excellent chance of recovery from her first episode, but also a strong likelihood of having another episode in the future. Her next episode will probably be a depressive episode, but another manic episode can occur at a later time.

Actions in your child's treatment that could delay or reduce the symptoms of the next episode include stress management, good sleep habits (lack of sleep is known to trigger mania), and avoidance of drugs or alcohol. Taking prescribed medicines is very important, but it doesn't necessarily prevent a recurrence, speaking to the fact that lifestyle can play a significant role in maintaining recovery. Ask your doctor how you, as a parent, can help your daughter avoid a future episode.

21. What are the chances that a child who is diagnosed with a mood disorder will kill himself or herself?

A review of adult studies on suicide conducted almost 40 years ago showed the rate of suicide in people with mood disorders to be 30 times the rate of the general population. The answer to this question as it relates to a child is rather complicated, since it depends on a number of factors unique to the child's situation. Rather than give a calculation of risk, I would prefer to discuss the issues and who is at risk. Certain members of the population are more likely to commit suicide than others. Older teens and young adults have a higher risk of suicide than school-aged children. Males kill themselves more often than females, although females try to commit suicide (without succeeding) three times more often than males. Members of certain ethnic groups have a dramatically higher risk for suicide than their counterparts, including Alaskan or Native American youth. Some adult studies show that up to 15% of those with Bipolar I disorder will commit suicide. Between the sexes, however, differences in risk are posed by the presence of a mood disorder. For girls, the presence of major depression raises the risk of suicide substantially higher than that of the general population, while for boys, a previous suicide attempt is associated with a higher risk of completing suicide. Other factors, such as the presence of a gun at home, parent-child conflict, use of drugs or alcohol at the time of suicide, a past history of abuse (especially sexual abuse), and parental psychiatric disorders also increase the risk of suicide in a youngster.

A parent whose child has been diagnosed with depression or bipolar disorder might be alarmed to hear these statistics about suicide. However, statistics also show that the majority of people who kill themselves were not in treatment. A child who is working with a doctor for his mood disorder has a lower risk profile for suicide than one who does not seek help. Also, the literature has shown that treatment lowers the risk of suicide associated with mood disorders.

There's no doubt that those afflicted with mood disorders have a high rate of suicide. Your child may have one or more characteristics that constitute risk, and that can be frightening. However, thinking and worrying about his chances of suicide based on larger statistics without regard for individual circumstances is not very helpful. Instead, it's probably far more useful to discuss with your doctor the specific risk factors particular to your child, and if possible aim to reduce some of those risks in treatment.

PART THREE

Diagnosis

What are the symptoms of depression in a child or adolescent?

What are the symptoms of bipolar disorder in children?

What other problems could be associated with a mood disorder?

How do you manage aggression?

More . . .

22. How are emotional problems diagnosed in children and adolescents? What guidelines will a doctor use in arriving at a diagnosis?

In the United States, doctors (usually psychiatrists) will use the *Diagnostic and Statistical Manual of Mental Disorders*, 4th Edition (*DSM*-IV, or commonly referred to as *DSM*) as the standard guide in classifying and diagnosing illnesses. Other countries may use the *DSM* or another manual system called the *International Classification of Disorders*, 10th Edition (*ICD*-10). In either case, the manual provides detailed descriptions and criteria that must be fulfilled in order to diagnose psychiatric disorders. The *DSM* and *ICD*-10 are important tools used to arrive at a diagnosis; however, they are most useful in the hands of someone who is experienced at applying the criteria.

The diagnosis of depression or BPD is not simply "plugging-in" symptoms into a check list. Rather, a doctor will arrive at a diagnosis using first the history provided by the child and her family, along with careful interview and observation of the child. Other pieces of information may also be needed to provide a well rounded view of the emotional problem, such as input from a teacher and other family members, and the degree of disability in the community caused by the problem. The clinical experience and intuition of the doctor will also guide what other questions to ask and observations to make. In addition to history taken from different sources, other tools in the diagnostic process may include the use of written questionnaires or standardized tests to elicit information that might not have come up during the interview. The assignment of a *DSM* diagnosis is usually the last part of the evaluation.

23. What are the symptoms of depression in a child or adolescent?

A child will almost never tell you, "I'm depressed." Instead, the power of observation and specific questioning of caregivers and other adults in the child's life will help identify the symptoms. The *DSM* describes three depressive disorders that reflect partial or full criteria for a major depressive episode (MDE). If you refer to Table 1, the criteria for an MDE are listed. As described, an MDE requires a prolonged, depressed mood or loss of pleasure in favorite activities for two weeks or more, and at least four other symptoms are needed to meet the diagnosis, along with other characteristics. The list of symptoms includes problems with sleep, weight or appetite changes, feelings of guilt, low energy, concentration problems, agitation or being slowed down, or suicidal thinking. In children and adolescents, a depressed mood might appear as irritability. Aggression such as fighting (physical aggression) or cursing/disrespectful talk (verbal aggression) can be a manifestation of irritability, or it could represent agitation. (More on aggression is discussed in Questions 32 and 38). Loss of pleasure in favorite activities could be seen as reduced amounts of play with toys, games, or usual playmates. Activities that usually light a spark in your child no longer hold much interest for him. Loss of pleasure could also be seen as detachment from family members or friends with whom the child is normally engaged. Preoccupation with sadness could be a theme in play rather than verbal statements of sadness. Disturbances of sleep may

The list of symptoms includes problems with sleep, weight or appetite changes, feelings of guilt, low energy, concentration problems, agitation or being slowed down, or suicidal thinking.

be observed as either an inability to sleep at night, or excessive sleeping, both of which are commonly noted among depressed teenagers. Concentration problems may be seen in the classroom or as the inability to do homework or other assignments. A decline in school performance noticed by a teacher or guidance counselor or poor marks on a report card may be an indicator of concentration problems. Major depressive disorder (MDD) describes having one or more major depressive episodes.

Table 1   Modified Criteria for a Major Depressive Episode

- **A depressed or irritable mood** most of the day, nearly every day, as indicated by either subjective report (e.g., feels sad or empty) or observation made by others (e.g., appears tearful)

  OR

  Markedly diminished interest or pleasure in all, or almost all, activities most of the day, nearly every day (as indicated by either subjective account or observation made by others)

  AND

  Four (or more) of the following symptoms have been present during the same 2-week period nearly every day and represent a change from previous functioning:
  - significant weight loss or gain, change in appetite, or failure to make expected weight gains
  - sleep problems
  - agitation or sluggishness
  - lack of energy
  - feelings of worthlessness or excessive guilt
  - concentration problems or indecision
  - recurrent thoughts of death (not just fear of dying), recurrent suicidal thoughts, a suicide attempt, or plan for committing suicide
- The symptoms cause **clinically significant distress or impairment** in social, occupational, or other important areas of functioning.
- The symptoms are **not due to the direct effect of drugs or illness**.
- The symptoms are **not due to bereavement**, unless it lasts longer than 2 months and has other complicated features.

(Adapted with permission from the *Diagnostic and Statistical Manual of Mental Disorders*, Text Revision, Fourth Edition. Copyright 2000. American Psychiatric Association.)

Once an MDE has been diagnosed, it is further defined as mild, moderate, or severe, and if either psychosis (hallucinations or delusions) is present, or if other unusual features exist. Mild depression usually refers to an MDE that fulfills fewer symptoms from the list of the criteria (e.g., 5–7 criteria) and a higher degree of functioning is observed. Severe depression usually refers to an MDE that fulfills nearly all the symptoms from the list of criteria (e.g., 7–9 criteria), often including **suicidality**, and/or an extremely low degree of functioning (e.g., the child can't attend school, stays in bed all day, has poor hygiene). Moderate depression describes an MDE that is between mild and moderate in terms of criteria and degree of functioning. The rating of mild, moderate, or severe for depression and the presence or absence of psychosis are important with regard to treatment options, further discussed in Questions 34, 46, and 63.

Suicidality

Suicidal thoughts, actions such as suicide attempts or other harmful behaviors that could lead to suicide.

24. Why is it called a "major depression"? Are there other kinds of depression? What does "clinical depression" mean?

The term "major depression" comes from the first definition of Major Depressive Disorder that appeared in an earlier edition of the *DSM* (the *DSM*-III, published in 1980). At that time, a "major feature" of the illness involved having a depressed mood, along with five criteria from a list similar to the one used in *DSM*-IV-TR. Nowadays, when we call a psychiatric condition "major depression" we are usually referring to an MDE or MDD. Other types of depression also exist in the current edition of the *DSM*. These include

Dysthymic disorder

Also known as "dysthymia." According to the *DSM*, dysthymic disorder is diagnosed in children and adolescents when a depressed or irritable mood is observed almost all the time for a year or more, and at least two symptoms drawing from the list for an MDE, as well as other features are also noted (see Table 7).

Clinical depression is generally synonymous with an MDE, MDD, or the depressive component of bipolar disorder, and it also suggests that treatment is needed.

Hypomania

Behavior that would fit the criteria for a hypomanic episode. A hypomanic episode is described in the *DSM* as a period of elevated or irritable mood for 4 days or more, along with other criteria (see Table 3).

dysthymic disorder, (see also Question 29), or a significant pattern of depressive symptoms that do not fit the diagnosis of MDD but cause some impairment, known as fepressive disorder NOS in the *DSM*. This last diagnosis may include a problem, referred to as "minor depressive disorder" in the *DSM*. The term "minor depressive disorder" describes a condition that draws from the same list as MDD, but includes only two to four criteria, rather than the five or more of MDD. That term is used infrequently now (it existed as an official diagnosis in the past, but no longer) and is used mainly for research purposes. The term "clinical depression" usually implies that a doctor or other "clinician" (someone who treats patients) should be involved in the care of an afflicted person. Clinical depression is generally synonymous with an MDE, MDD, or the depressive component of bipolar disorder, and it also suggests that treatment is needed.

25. What are the symptoms of bipolar disorder in children?

Bipolar disorder (BPD) is a psychiatric illness that is characterized by one or more episodes of mania or hypomania (see Tables 2 and 3), and possibly also major depressive episodes. It is also known as manic-depressive illness, or manic-depression. The two common types of BPD are Bipolar I Disorder, where the person experiences manic episodes alone or mixed with depression, and a milder version, Bipolar II Disorder, where the person experiences **hypomania** and major depressive episodes. BPD is generally cyclical in nature, which means that the person experiencing it fluctuates between episodes of mania, hypomania, depression, or a combination of these problems.

Table 2   Modified Criteria for a Manic Episode

- A distinct period of abnormally and persistently **elevated, expansive, or irritable mood**, lasting at least **1 week** (or any duration if hospitalization is necessary).
- During this period, **three (or more) of the following symptoms** have persisted (four if the mood is only irritable) and have been present to a significant degree:
  - inflated self-esteem or grandiosity
  - decreased need for sleep (e.g., feels rested after only 3 hours of sleep)
  - excessive speech or pressured speech
  - racing thoughts
  - distractibility
  - increase in goal-directed activity (either socially, at work or school, or sexually) or agitation
  - excessive involvement in pleasurable activities that have a high potential for painful consequences (e.g., engaging in unrestrained buying sprees, sexual indiscretions, or foolish business investments)
- There is marked **impairment** in occupational **functioning** or in usual social activities or relationships with others, hospitalization to prevent harm to self or others is necessary, or there are psychotic features.
- The symptoms are **not due to the direct effects of drugs, illness, or antidepressant treatments**.

(Modified from the *DSM*-IV TR, Washington, DC, American Psychiatric Association.)

26. What is mania?

Mania is a term used by professionals to describe a manic episode. The *DSM* defines a manic episode as a period of irritable, elevated, or expansive mood lasting 1 week or more, that is accompanied by three or more symptoms from a list of other possible criteria (see Table 2). These include a reduced need for sleep, increased risk-taking behaviors, a change in speech known as "pressured speech" (talking more quickly, in larger amounts), and increased hyperactivity. More often than not, children and adolescents present with irritability rather than the elevated mood.

Table 3   Modified Criteria for a Hypomanic Episode

- A distinct period of persistently **elevated, expansive, or irritable mood**, lasting throughout at least **4 days**, that is clearly different from the usual nondepressed mood

  AND

  During this period, **three (or more)** of the symptoms listed for a manic episode have persisted (four if the mood is only irritable) and have been present to a significant degree.

- The episode represents a change in functioning that is uncharacteristic of the person when not symptomatic. See Table 2 for the list of symptoms for a manic episode.

- The disturbance in mood and the **change in functioning** are observable by others.

- The episode is **not severe enough to cause marked impairment** in social or occupational functioning, or to necessitate hospitalization, and there are no psychotic features.

- The symptoms are **not due to the direct effects of drugs, illness, or antidepressant treatments**.

(Adapted with permission from the *Diagnostic and Statistical Manual of Mental Disorders*, Text Revision, Fourth Edition. Copyright 2000. American Psychiatric Association.)

Episodes of mania that occur for intervals of time shorter than a week are referred to as "hypomania," generally 4 days to a week (see Table 3). Even more frequent fluctuations of manic symptoms can be observed (hours or even a couple of days). This phenomenon is known as cyclothymic disorder or "cyclothymia" in the *DSM* (see Table 6).

The *DSM* describes a pattern of BPD as "rapid cycling," when mood episodes (either depression, mania, or both) occurs more than four times a year. Other possible patterns of either MDD or BPD include the presence or absence of full recovery of symptoms between episodes, or the occurrence of depressive or manic episodes at certain times of year. In the latter case, the episodes are described to have a seasonal pattern. An example of a mood disorder with a seasonal pattern is seasonal affective disorder (SAD), also known as winter depression, a term not found in the *DSM* but commonly understood by scientists as a disorder with recurrent major depressive episodes occurring in the winter months.

In order to have Bipolar I Disorder, the child must have had at least one manic episode or a mixed episode consisting of manic and depressive symptoms in his lifetime. At other times, major depressive episodes may occur alone, alternate with, or occur concurrently with episodes of mania. When depression occurs at the same time as mania, the episode of illness is called a "mixed episode" (see Table 4). Those who experience the shorter, less severe episodes of hypomania are classified as having Bipolar II Disorder (see Table 5), whereas those who have the typical 1-week episode of mania, have Bipolar I Disorder.

Table 4   Modified Criteria for a Mixed Episode

- Criteria are met both for a manic episode and for a major depressive episode nearly every day during at least a 1-week period.
- There is marked **impairment** in occupational functioning or in usual social activities or relationships with others, hospitalization to prevent harm to self or others is necessary, or there are psychotic features.
- The symptoms are **not due to the direct effects of drugs, illness, or antidepressant treatments**.

(Adapted with permission from the *Diagnostic and Statistical Manual of Mental Disorders*, Text Revision, Fourth Edition. Copyright 2000. American Psychiatric Association.)

Table 5   Modified Diagnostic Criteria for Bipolar II Disorder

- There is at least one **major depressive episode**.
- There is at least one **hypomanic episode.**
- There are no manic or mixed episodes.
- Symptoms are not better accounted for by a psychotic disorder.
- Symptoms cause clinically **significant distress or impairment** in social, occupational, or other important areas of functioning.

(Adapted with permission from the *Diagnostic and Statistical Manual of Mental Disorders*, Text Revision, Fourth Edition. Copyright 2000. American Psychiatric Association.)

Table 6 Modified Diagnostic Criteria for Cyclothymic Disorder in Children and Adolescents

- For at least **1 year**, there has been presence of **numerous periods with hypomanic symptoms and numerous periods with depressive symptoms**.
- During this 1-year period, the person has not been symptom-free for more than 2 months at a time.
- No major depressive episode, manic episode, or mixed episode has been present during the first year of the disturbance.
- The symptoms are not better accounted for by a psychotic disorder.
- The symptoms are **not due to the direct effects of drugs or illness**.
- The symptoms cause **significant distress or impairment** in social, occupational, or other important areas of functioning.

(Adapted with permission from the *Diagnostic and Statistical Manual of Mental Disorders*, Text Revision, Fourth Edition. Copyright 2000. American Psychiatric Association.)

Regardless of the specific symptoms or subtype of BPD your child may have, the treatment approaches to the problems are generally the same.

Regardless of the specific symptoms or subtype of BPD your child may have, the treatment approaches to the problems are generally the same. For this reason, many professionals will not call the illness by its subtype, but just "bipolar disorder." People who have BPD will often call themselves, "bipolar."

27. What is the difference between "unipolar" and "bipolar" depression?

Unipolar depression refers to what we usually think of when we hear about depression—an MDE, MDD, or other types of depressive disorder without mania or hypomania. If a child is experiencing unipolar depression, she no longer qualifies for BPD. "Bipolar" depression refers to depression that is part of the larger cycle of BPD. As mentioned previously, bipolar depression occurs before, after, or during an episode of mania. The two terms, unipolar and bipolar depression, essentially distinguish to other professionals whether a child has MDD versus BPD.

28. My daughter was diagnosed with an "adjustment disorder"—what is that?

According to the *DSM*, an adjustment disorder is a time-limited condition that occurs within 3 months of a stressful event, and is characterized by either distress or impairment in functioning. The condition resolves within 6 months of the stressful event, and is not part of bereavement. Adjustment disorders have symptoms that may include depression, anxiety, conduct problems, or a combination of these features (see Table 7 for the diagnostic criteria for an adjustment disorder). The symptoms of suicidal thoughts or attempts are

---

Table 7   Modified Diagnostic Criteria for Adjustment Disorders

- The development of **emotional or behavioral symptoms** in response to an identifiable stressor(s) occurring **within 3 months** of the onset of the stressor(s).
- These symptoms or behaviors are clinically significant as evidenced by either of the following:
  - distress in excess of what would be expected from exposure to the stressor
  - significant impairment in social or occupational (academic) functioning
- The stress-related disturbance is not due to another diagnosis or bereavement.
- Once the stressor is gone, the symptoms remit within 6 months.

Adjustment disorders are classified by the following types:
- With depressed mood
- With mixed anxiety and depressed mood
- With anxiety
- With disturbance of conduct
- With mixed disturbance of emotions and conduct
- Unspecified

(Adapted with permission from the *Diagnostic and Statistical Manual of Mental Disorders*, Text Revision, Fourth Edition. Copyright 2000. American Psychiatric Association.)

absent in an adjustment disorder. Professionals feel that an adjustment disorder carries a better prognosis than a mood or anxiety disorder. An adjustment disorder may respond to non-pharmacologic (non-medication) therapies more easily than MDD.

29. What is dysthymic disorder? What is a "double depression"?

Dysthymic disorder or "dysthymia" is a low grade, more continuous state of depression (see Table 8). It lasts much longer than an MDE (which generally resolves over a number of months), in this case for at

---

Table 8   Modified Diagnostic Criteria for Dysthymic Disorder in Children and Adolescents

- **Depressed or irritable mood** is present for most of the day, nearly every day for **at least 1 year**.
- **Two (or more)** of the following:
  - poor appetite or overeating
  - insomnia or hypersomnia
  - low energy or fatigue
  - low self-esteem
  - poor concentration or difficulty making decisions
  - feelings of hopelessness
- During the 1-year period of the disturbance, the person has never been symptom-free for more than 2 months at a time.
- No other depressive disorders have been present during the first year of the disturbance.
- There has never been a manic episode, a mixed episode, a hypo-manic episode, or cyclothymic disorder.
- The disturbance does not occur during the course of a psychotic disorder.
- The symptoms are **not due to the direct effects of drugs or illness**.
- The symptoms cause clinically significant distress or **impairment** in social, occupational, or other important areas of functioning.

(Adapted with permission from the *Diagnostic and Statistical Manual of Mental Disorders*, Text Revision, Fourth Edition. Copyright 2000. American Psychiatric Association.)

least 1 year in children and adolescents, and 2 years or more in adults. A "double depression" is the condition named by professionals of a new MDE superimposed on a baseline of dysthymia. It is not a *DSM* term, but would appear as two diagnoses (MDD and dysthymia) if the *DSM* were used to describe the condition.

30. What other problems could be associated with a mood disorder?

Other problems frequently occur at the same time as either MDD or BPD. These are known as comorbid conditions or comorbidities. They may include anxiety disorders, drug or alcohol problems, learning problems, disruptive disorders such as attention deficit hyperactivity disorder (ADHD), behaviors that involve trouble with the law, and several other difficulties. At times, the comorbid disorder may have taken place before the diagnosis of a mood disorder was made. At other times, the comorbidity occurs at the same time or well after the mood disorder has been established.

The implication in having more than one diagnosis is that the treatment is usually more complicated. Different psychotherapies or medications are probably indicated to address these situations. School interventions such as working with the local Committee on Special Education (CSE) or its equivalent to identify educational resources to help with your child's academic progress may also be needed. Sometimes legal interventions and/or substance abuse programming may be required as well to handle the complicated treatment demands of having a mood disorder and comorbidity.

When the mood disorder is treated effectively, it may prevent or improve a comorbid disorder. An example of such a case would be one where good control of mania or depression is achieved, which may then prevent a youngster from needing to use drugs or alcohol to tolerate the symptoms during manic or depressive episodes. Another example may be one where a learning-disordered bipolar child with appropriate educational resources and management may experience less overall stress and depressive symptoms.

You should consult with your doctor about how you and your child can navigate the challenges faced with living with both a mood disorder and another emotional disorder. Family support organizations such as those mentioned in Question 100 can also be very helpful for those with comorbid illnesses.

Geraldine's comment:

With regards to school interventions, the Committee on Special Education in our school district suggested a smaller class for our daughter, Lexie. Unfortunately, the placement they recommended had kids with autism and learning disabilities, which didn't seem like the right fit for my child who had neither of these problems, although it had the right ratio of children to teachers. A continued dialogue with educators was needed to help Lexie obtain the right placement. At one point, we saw a psychiatrist who wanted to observe our child in school to help advocate for the correct placement. It was difficult to have to sit through a lot of evaluations and meetings to achieve the right balance in educational environment. Ultimately, she was placed in a classroom in public school that operates like a day treatment, with an intensive level of supervision for the group of children who all have emotional problems.

Our son has always gotten a lot of support in school, but it's required our constant involvement. Just last year, he finally got services to help with his writing after educators found him to have a learning disorder with regards to writing.

31. My son was diagnosed and treated for ADHD by his pediatrician when he was in the first grade. Now that he is older, a different doctor says he has bipolar disorder. Which is the correct diagnosis?

You are describing a classic problem in the diagnosis of children and adolescents: at one developmental stage, he receives one diagnosis and, at a later stage, he gets a completely different one. Your son is not alone in having received the diagnoses of ADHD and BPD. At one time it was thought that a child could have one but not the other, and it was a matter of correctly differentiating symptoms common to both disorders such as hyperactivity and poor impulse control. Table 9 on ADHD will reveal the *DSM* criteria for this disorder. Furthermore, the presentation of symptoms are often vague and diffuse in early-onset BPD, and irritability and sleep problems are very common in ADHD (even though they are not on the list of *DSM* criteria). These types of situations could lead to misdiagnosis in some patients. Experts on BPD indicate that some symptoms, such as grandiosity and reduced need for sleep, could be more suggestive of BPD over ADHD, but it remains a debated area among child psychiatrists. Recent research shows that a surprisingly high number

Table 9   Modified Diagnostic Criteria for Attention-Deficit/Hyperactivity Disorder (ADHD)

Six (or more) symptoms of **inattention or hyperactivity-impulsivity** for at least 6 months to a degree that is maladaptive and inconsistent with developmental level (see Symptom Criteria for ADHD listed below), and:

- symptoms were present before age 7 years
- impairment is present in two or more settings (e.g., at school [or work] and at home)
- evidence of significant impairment in social, academic, or occupational functioning is noted
- symptoms are not better accounted for by another mental disorder

Types of ADHD:
- Attention-deficit/hyperactivity disorder, *combined type*: if both inattentive criteria and hyperactive-impulsive criteria are fulfilled
- Attention-deficit/hyperactivity disorder, *predominantly inattentive type*: if only inattentive criteria are fulfilled
- Attention-deficit/hyperactivity disorder, *predominantly hyperactive-impulsive type*: if only hyperactive-impulsive criteria are fulfilled

Symptom Criteria for ADHD:
Inattention
- often fails to give close attention to details or makes careless mistakes in schoolwork, work, or other activities
- often has difficulty sustaining attention in tasks or play activities
- often does not seem to listen when spoken to directly
- often does not follow through on instructions and fails to finish schoolwork, chores, or duties in the workplace (not due to oppositional behavior or failure to understand instructions)
- often has difficulty organizing tasks and activities
- often avoids, dislikes, or is reluctant to engage in tasks that require sustained mental effort (such as schoolwork or homework)
- often loses things necessary for tasks or activities (e.g., toys, school assignments, pencils, books, or tools)
- is often easily distracted by extraneous stimuli
- is often forgetful in daily activities

Hyperactivity
- often fidgets with hands or feet, or squirms in seat
- often leaves seat in classroom or in other situations in which remaining seated is expected
- often runs about or climbs excessively in inappropriate situations (in adolescents or adults, may be limited to subjective feelings of restlessness)
- often has difficulty playing or engaging in leisure activities quietly
- is often "on the go" or often acts as if "driven by a motor"
- often talks excessively

Impulsivity
- often blurts out answers before questions have been completed
- often has difficulty awaiting turn
- often interrupts or intrudes on others (e.g., butts into conversations or games)

(Adapted with permission from the *Diagnostic and Statistical Manual of Mental Disorders*, Text Revision, Fourth Edition. Copyright 2000. American Psychiatric Association.)

of patients can have symptoms of both ADHD and BPD, and that it is not unusual to carry both diagnoses. These patients are often treated using a combination of therapies that address symptoms for each of the disorders (see Table 10 for a list of ADHD medications). One of the reasons that ADHD is often an earlier diagnosis in children has to do with the earlier presentation of disruptive symptoms in preschool and elementary school. Mood disorders generally don't start at that age, and thus the diagnosis of ADHD is often considered more frequently during this period.

Table 10   Medications Used to Treat ADHD

Generic Name	Brand Name
Stimulants	
Methylphenidate	Methylin, Methylin ER tablets
	Ritalin tablets, Ritalin LA capsules, Ritalin SR tablets
	Metadate ER tablets, Metadate CD capsules
	Focalin, Focalin XR tablets
	Daytrana patch
	Concerta tablets
Amphetamine	Dexedrine, Dextrostat tablets, Dexedrine spansules/capsules
	Adderall tablets, Adderall XR capsules
	Vyvanse tablets
Norepinephrine Reuptake Inhibitor (NRI)	
Atomoxetine	Strattera
Blood Pressure Medications (Alpha adrenergic agonists)	
Clonidine	Catapres
Guanfacine	Tenex
Norepinephrine Dopamine Reuptake Inhibitor (NDRI)	
Buproprion	Wellbutrin, Wellbutrin SR, Wellbutrin XL
Tricyclic Antidepressants (TCAs)	
Nortriptyline	Pamelor, Aventyl
Imipramine	Tofranil, Tofranil-PM
Desipramine	Norpramin

As a parent, it can be unsettling to see your son receiving different diagnoses, and even more so if he may need to take multiple medications for his behavior. It will be important to review with your current doctor what symptoms he attributes to BPD, and if any residual ADHD symptoms exist that may need attention. Also, the prior response to ADHD medications, such as **psychostimulants** should be discussed, since an inadequate response might suggest that the symptoms represented **prodromal** (early stage or the stage just before the diagnosis of) BPD. A good response might indicate future consideration in the treatment of the current condition(s). You will also need to communicate with your pediatrician, if you haven't already, about any changes in the presentation of your son's illness that have led to a revised diagnosis of BPD.

Geraldine's comment:

Our family knows all too well what it's like to experience multiple diagnoses. In the case of both our children, symptoms of ADHD and depressive disorders have occurred. What's more, it's easy to see how having one behavioral problem like ADHD over time can lead to other problems. Our son, Joseph, started out with ADHD symptoms but now that he's 11, the low self-esteem and low mood associated with having these symptoms uncontrolled for such a long time has become apparent. He thinks he's always going to get in trouble in school and that the teacher doesn't like him, even though that isn't the case at all. When he gets a bad grade on a test, he really blames himself for not having done a better job.

Psychostimulants

Also known as "stimulants." Medications that increase the brain's alertness, hence the name. Two major categories of psychostimulants include methylphenidate and amphetamine. This group of medications is used to treat ADHD as well as a problem with wakefulness known as narcolepsy.

Prodromal stage

A period of time before diagnosis of an illness such as bipolar disorder or a psychotic disorder, when symptoms exist but are much more subtle and not yet causing disability. The period can exist for months or years before the illness fully presents.

32. My daughter is very aggressive. Why is she like this when my wife and I are not this way at home?

Parents feel very guilty or embarrassed when their child behaves in a way in public that is different from what is taught or modeled at home. Verbal and physical aggression are definitely behaviors that can be learned from disturbed adults who are exposing their children to such things. Yet, most parents don't subject their children to violence. In children, aggressive behavior can be a nonspecific symptom of what they are experiencing, rather than an imitation of something seen at home. Aggression could be a child's way of reacting to an internal state such as depression, anxiety, or irritability. Mood disorders commonly present with symptoms of aggression. Children are especially susceptible to aggressive behavior, for the important reason that they are often less able to use words to express how they're doing as compared to actions. The reason for this is often due to the fact that cognitive development (in this case in the form of communication) takes longer to mature than does physical development. Also, the ability to solve conflicts in a socially appropriate manner is a skill that takes time to develop.

Other causes of aggression exist. Children can also react to stressors at home such as marital conflict between parents, or to major family crises such as a death of a loved one or other losses. Other causes of aggression in children and adolescents could include having been assaulted, abused or using drugs. Children who witnessed or experienced violence can also show signs of aggressive behavior. In these cases, they may have learned the behaviors or they may be "playing out" the violence (mental health professionals call it

Parents feel very guilty or embarrassed when their child behaves in a way in public that is different from what is taught or modeled at home.

Diagnosis

re-enactment of the trauma) previously witnessed as a way for them to get through the experience of anger, fear, and confusion felt as the witness. Traumatized children may also be aggressive as part of a disorder known as **post-traumatic stress disorder (PTSD)** (see Table 11), where the aggression represents a type of hyper-reactivity known as hypervigilance. Children who are undergoing a major change in their routine or environment, such as starting a new school, can experience a tremendous amount of stress and exhibit increased amounts of irritability, which can lead to aggression in some cases. Finally, children with developmental delays such as language delays or autism, commonly present with aggression as a means of conveying frustration that the child is unable to verbalize or solving problems in more immature ways. The case of your child needs to be further evaluated by your doctor in order to better understand the reasons for the violent behavior.

Going back to the question previously raised, sometimes parents and other caregivers may not realize the impact they have on their child's behavior. Adults in every child's life need to be aware of their own actions, and how behaviors such as a using a harsh voice tone most of the time, arguing, cursing, and obviously engaging in threats and violence, can have a negative impact on a developing child's emotional state. Even if your child is diagnosed with a mood disorder, he is still like other children in the sense that what you do will have an influence on him. Parents often forget that what they do at home is constantly being taken in by their children. Often, self-reflection is needed on the part of parents, to better understand how you and other adult caregivers are modeling behaviors for your child. If you have any problems in that area, don't hesi-

Post-Traumatic Stress Disorder

Also known as "PTSD." This is a *DSM* disorder that is characterized by groups of symptoms that include hyperarousal, avoidance, and reexperiencing an event after having been exposed to a life-threatening or harmful event. More details about PTSD are described in Table 11.

Parents often forget that what they do at home is constantly being taken in by their children.

Table 11   Modified Diagnostic Criteria for Post-Traumatic Stress Disorder (PTSD) in Children

- The person has been exposed to a traumatic event in which the threat of death or serious harm was present, and the person was fearful, helpless, horrified, disorganized, or agitated.
- The traumatic event is persistently reexperienced in one (or more) of the following ways:
  - recurrent and intrusive distressing recollections of the event, including images, thoughts, or perceptions. *Note*: In young children, repetitive play may occur in which themes or aspects of the trauma are expressed.
  - recurrent distressing dreams of the event. *Note*: In children, there may be frightening dreams without recognizable content.
  - acting or feeling as if the traumatic event were recurring (includes a sense of reliving the experience, illusions, hallucinations, and dissociative flashback episodes, including those that occur on awakening or when intoxicated). *Note*: In young children, trauma-specific reenactment may occur.
  - intense psychological distress at exposure to internal or external cues that symbolize or resemble an aspect of the traumatic event
  - physiological reactivity on exposure to internal or external cues that symbolize or resemble an aspect of the traumatic event
- Persistent avoidance of stimuli associated with the trauma and numbing of general responsiveness (not present before the trauma), as indicated by three (or more) of the following:
  - efforts to avoid thoughts, feelings, or conversations associated with the trauma
  - efforts to avoid activities, places, or people that arouse recollections of the trauma
  - inability to recall an important aspect of the trauma
  - markedly diminished interest or participation in significant activities
  - feeling of detachment or estrangement from others
  - restricted range of affect (e.g., unable to have loving feelings)
  - sense of a foreshortened future (e.g., does not expect to have a career, marriage, children, or a normal life span)
- Persistent symptoms of increased arousal (not present before the trauma), as indicated by two (or more) of the following:
  - difficulty falling or staying asleep
  - irritability or outbursts of anger
  - difficulty concentrating
  - hypervigilance
  - exaggerated startle response
- Duration of the disturbance is more than 1 month.
- The disturbance causes clinically significant distress or impairment in social, occupational, or other important areas of functioning.
- The disturbance can be acute if less than 3 months or chronic if 3 months or more

(Adapted with permission from the *Diagnostic and Statistical Manual of Mental Disorders*, Text Revision, Fourth Edition. Copyright 2000. American Psychiatric Association.)

Diagnosis

55

tate to get help for them yourself. Remember, helping yourself is actually helping your child by making you a better parent.

The management of aggression is further discussed in Question 38.

33. Are other parts of the body affected when a child is depressed?

The body, along with the mind, often expresses itself. Headaches, stomachaches, and other aches and pains commonly occur in children who are depressed or anxious. School-aged children (those between 5 and 12) are frequent sufferers of these types of bodily complaints that could be part of depression, or even normal levels of anxiety. These problems should not be discounted or ignored, however, as coming only from their heads. When they first present, they should always be evaluated first by your pediatrician to ensure that treatable medical conditions have not occurred. Some common medical problems in children such as lactose intolerance, acid reflux disease, or constipation, could all cause stomachaches, and require medical management. Similarly, a migraine headache or, less commonly, a brain tumor could cause headaches and need attention from your pediatrician. If your primary care doctor finds no physical basis for the complaints, they should still be taken seriously, since they can cause significant impairment in functioning. Often, a child is seeking reassurance for other emotional needs when she is presenting with a physical complaint, and denying that it is real can only make the child feel worse. A different approach in the form of a specialized behavioral plan for the child may be needed if the aches and pains are causing her to spend too much time in the school nurse's office, out of class, or otherwise avoiding other important activities such as attending class or taking a test. This type of plan is best made with you, your doctor, and other adults such as teachers after your pediatrician has done the initial evaluation of the complaints.

34. My child is depressed and hears voices. How can I be sure that my child does not have schizophrenia?

Hallucinations (hearing voices or seeing things that are not there) and other breaks in reality which include excessive, unfounded suspicion (paranoia), false beliefs (delusions), or odd, disorganized behavior are generally known as psychotic experiences or psychosis. These are often what come to mind when thinking about mental illness and can be very scary, and concerning to both the child and his family. Psychosis is common to several conditions such as schizophrenia, major depressive disorder with psychotic features, bipolar disorder, or substance abuse. Only your doctor can clarify the underlying condition causing these experiences. At times, the diagnosis of the problem can be challenging. However, depression with hallucinations is far more common in children than schizophrenia. Furthermore, schizophrenia presents with other problems of severe social and occupational/academic dysfunction. Often, children with schizophrenia may have had other, subtle developmental problems since early childhood. Some parents find that they have always known their child to be different than others from an early age. The history of your child's emotional development, as well as the current presentation of illness, will inform your doctor as to the diagnosis. Still, bipolar disorder in childhood has been confused with schizophrenia by novice and skilled clinicians alike, as the presentations are so similar, and time to mature further is sometimes needed before a more certain diagnosis is attained. Parents can be understandably worried about schizophrenia, since it often has a poorer prognosis than a depressive or bipolar disorder. In most cases, time will tell as to which disorder is affecting your child. Again, it is imperative that these concerns be raised with your child's doctor, so that clarifications can be made.

35. What medical evaluations will be needed once my child is diagnosed with a mood disorder?

Your child's psychiatrist will most likely want a thorough medical evaluation of your child, including blood and urine tests. Your pediatrician may be asked to perform some or all of these tests, or you may be asked to obtain some of the tests directly through a laboratory. One of the reasons for such extensive evaluation is that, occasionally, correctable medical problems may cause symptoms of a mood disorder (see also Question 37). In such cases, it would not be appropriate to assume that psychotherapy and/or psychiatric medications alone would treat the disorder. One example of this is hypothyroidism, where a child may gain weight, look and appear lethargic, and have a depressed mood. The problem is one of low production of an important hormone called thyroid hormone. Once the cause of the deficiency has been determined, the treatment is to replace the missing hormone. This can often result in an improvement in the symptoms.

The first part of the medical evaluation is a physical examination, including height and weight, to determine your child's physical health. Blood tests are frequently requested. These include a complete blood count, blood chemistries, thyroid function tests, and possibly other tests. These tests are important to see that your child's organs such as the liver, kidneys, and bone marrow are functioning normally. Urine tests may also be done to check for normal kidney functioning, and for possible drug abuse. A test of heart functioning known as an electrocardiogram (EKG) may be requested to ensure that your child has a normal heart. If a decision to prescribe medications is made, your psychiatrist may be interested in following your child's height, weight, and certain other tests mentioned. This is done to monitor for any changes that may be caused by medications. Your psychiatrist may perform some of these tests herself, or she may work closely with your pediatrician to arrange for the tests.

These tests are important to see that your child's organs such as the liver, kidneys, and bone marrow are functioning normally.

36. Will my daughter's psychiatrist need to speak with anyone else about her depression?

With your permission, your doctor may want to speak with your child's teacher at school to find out more of what happens during the day with your child's behavior. Your child's teacher will know how she is doing in class, and if there are problems to be concerned about. A school guidance counselor or, if available, a school social worker may also be contacted. The opinions of any other staff from after-school programs may also be necessary. The perspectives of other adults in your child's life are important during the initial evaluation part of the treatment, and also during the treatment to assess how your child is responding to the treatment. If your child sees both a therapist and a psychiatrist, both providers will want to keep in close contact with each other.

Your child's psychiatrist may also want to be in touch with your child's pediatrician and review previous medical information to make certain that no medical problems or abnormal medical symptoms arise during the treatment period with medications.

Finally, and probably most important of all, the psychiatrist may want to meet or speak with one or both of the parents to obtain additional history about the problem, and address any ongoing concerns at home. Sometimes the doctor will even see parents without the child in order to gain a thorough history of the child's early years and more recent ones. Also, the relationship of the child with her parents is an important part of the assessment and treatment.

Some families don't want teachers and other "outsiders" in the child's life to be involved in his treatment. They may have concerns about the child's self-esteem, perception among friends and school personnel, or possible biases in how the child is treated that could occur as a result of sharing personal psychiatric information. As with any medical condition, information about a psychiatric condition is considered health information that is protected by law, and families are under no obligation to share this information with others in the community. Further discussion with your doctor will determine how important it will be to share psychiatric information with others not directly involved in the treatment. I would strongly suggest, however, that your child's pediatrician be among those aware and possibly included in the treatment, particularly if medications are being used. Primary care doctors are generally important partners in children's health and recovery from illnesses, whether medical or psychiatric.

Geraldine's comment:
One of the ways we knew that Lexie was responding to medication was by her teachers reporting an improvement in her ability to participate in class. Otherwise, it was not that obvious to us that she was any different. You need to consider the larger picture and all the adults involved in order to know if a treatment is a success or not.

37. Are there any medical illnesses that cause depression or mania?

Yes, although they are infrequent in children. It is hard to say whether the medical problem causes or is merely associated with the psychiatric symptoms. Often, if the medical problem is correctable, then once corrected, the mood symptoms disappear. Low thyroid hormone was already mentioned as one possible cause/association. In fact, low or high amounts of several other hormones produced by the body can also cause symptoms of a mood disorder. Other culprits include abnormal blood chemistries such as low calcium, anemia (low amount of red blood cells), high or low white blood cell count, and a number of other abnormalities. Infectious diseases can be associated with mood symptoms, including infection with the human immunodeficiency virus (HIV), Epstein Barr virus (EBV—the cause of "mono" or infectious mononucleosis), or Hepatitis B virus. Nutritional problems such as vitamin deficiency or excess have been implicated in mood symptoms. Other possible causes of mood problems include a certain type of seizure disorder, lead poisoning, or exacerbation of a chronic illness called Lupus. Some medications used to treat other medical problems can cause changes in mood, such as steroid treatment for asthma, chemotherapy drugs for cancer, or HIV medications.

The examples named here are only a few of the many possible causes of depressive, manic, or psychotic symptoms in children and adolescents. Further clarification with your doctor will determine if any of these other conditions may be the cause of your child's mood symptoms.

38. How do you manage aggression?

Aggression can be managed successfully, but it usually requires the participation of the patient, the parent(s), and the therapist and/or doctor. Some of the management occurs at home, and some can occur in the office of the doctor or therapist. The training and treatment philosophy of your mental health professional will reflect varying approaches to this problem. However, most likely, your mental health professional will recommend some combination of the following techniques.

First, the aggressive behavior must be identified by the family as "out of bounds" or totally inappropriate and unacceptable. Your child must understand this, or get help to understand it. The effect of your child's violence on the other person who was targeted must also be understood.

Next, the events that led up to violence need to be sorted out. What thoughts or feelings did your child experience just before he hit someone? Was there a misunderstanding or a disagreement that your child couldn't tolerate without losing control? What actually precipitated the event? Encourage your child to talk about what happened or have him tell you through other means like drawing about it or telling it as a story.

Explore with your child different strategies that he could use in a similar situation that are more adaptive than aggression. Help your child learn self-soothing techniques such as taking a walk, deep breathing, counting, drawing, or any number of other options to use in the face of frustration. Try to rehearse alternate outcomes such as in a role play between you and your child, re-enacting the situation that ended in violence. Younger children may find it helpful to use toys or puppets in play to express the situation. See if you can help your child come up with better solutions to the problem encountered than becoming aggressive.

Punish the aggression. Violent behavior should never be tolerated by the family and it needs to have consequences, regardless of how old your child is. The degree of punishment should be reflected by the severity of the action. For example, throwing or breaking things should have less of a penalty than hurting another person physically. Also, the type of punishment needs to be age-appropriate: giving a 12-year-old a time out doesn't work, nor does cancelling a trip to the movies work for a 3-year-old. Immediate consequences for inappropriate behavior can include reduction or elimination of allowance or other incentives (toys, clothing, etc.). Other possibilities include loss of privileges such as viewing television, use of electronic equipment, cell phones, etc. If the behavior happens in school, consequences determined by the educational system include suspension, and possibly expulsion.

Other management strategies for aggression affecting school behavior include placement in an alternate educational environment, usually achieved through the special education component of the public school system or through the private school sector that serves students with special needs. A smaller class size with more teaching staff is helpful for some children who become aggressive and inappropriate in a much larger setting. Some families, however, worry that being in such a class, often with other children that exhibit inappropriate behavior, could negatively influence their own child's conduct, or fail to provide the child with adequate academic stimulation. Also, many families and professionals believe that keeping their mood disordered child in a mainstream class can help from a social standpoint, and maintain some normalcy in their child's life which has otherwise been disrupted. The child should to be able to function academically in the larger class setting in order to benefit from this kind of arrangement. Further discussion with the teacher and school professionals should help clarify the child's needs, and whether changing the class is indicated. Question 40 also provides more information on specialized services in school.

You may want further guidance in some of these recommendations, which can be discussed with your doctor. In certain cases, more help, in the form of medication, will be required to treat the aggression. If the aggression is part of a larger problem, such as a manic episode of bipolar disorder, your doctor may choose to use antipsychotic and/or mood stabilizing medication, to supplement non-pharmacologic approaches being used at home and in treatment. Sometimes medications for depression or ADHD, such as the antidepressants or psychostimulants, can help with aggression by reducing the irritable mood or impulsivity which previously led to aggression. Severe violence may require prompt use of medications, a visit to a psychiatric emergency room, or possibly hospitalization.

39. I think my teenager is abusing drugs. Can this be the cause of his behavior problems?

If a youngster presents with a decline in school or social functioning, irritability, or unpredictable behavior, substance abuse could be the cause or a contributing factor. Other clues to drug abuse include a need for large amounts of money, lying, a change in hygiene or appearance, or a change in friends or peer group. Some drugs, such as cocaine, "crack," or alcohol, can cause a severe depressive reaction when the euphoric effects are wearing off. Teenagers, especially, can become suicidal, at risk for death or injury under these circumstances. The thinking process and judgment are quite impaired when under the influence and dangerous decisions such as reckless behavior (driving drunk or having unprotected sex) or violence could occur in these cases.

Some drugs, such as cocaine, "crack," or alcohol, can cause a severe depressive reaction when the euphoric effects are wearing off.

Some teenagers become involved with drugs simply out of boredom, for lack of being occupied with positive activities, or due to peer pressure. It's not uncommon for youngsters who are left on their own after school without a supervised or structured situation (formerly known as "latchkey" children) to venture out and befriend peers who are similarly unsupervised and get into unhealthy situations involving drugs. However, more often than not, the lack of supervision is the not the only reason for drug use; children may turn to drugs when they are experiencing painful or intolerable feelings along with having open time. Youth experiencing certain emotional problems are more likely to initiate substance abuse than the general population of youngsters. Recent statistics from the Substance Abuse Mental Health Service Administration (SAMHSA) reveal that youngsters with MDD are twice as likely to start using illicit drugs as compared with those who do not have the disorder. Certain symptoms, such as anxiety or hopelessness, could cause your son to use and possibly abuse marijuana or alcohol. Irritability or restlessness could cause him to abuse prescription drugs like painkillers which "slow down" the body and mind. A history of traumatic events such as sexual abuse, in particular, may predispose a young person to abuse drugs. A combination of factors, such as a serious personal loss such as the death of a close family member, desperate situations such as the loss of housing, financial troubles for the family, parental conflict, or other concerns, can also contribute to a teenager getting involved with drugs.

Talking to your son about drugs is a good idea. It's also very hard to do, since it is an awkward topic (like sex) to discuss between parents and children. It is even harder to have this kind of dialogue because many teenagers are not that talkative with their parents.

However, it really important to let your son know that it's okay to talk about it. Maybe he would be relieved to hear that you want to know how he's doing and that you would like to help him. He may be angry or in denial that there is problem. Regardless of the reaction, a discussion should occur. You may choose to involve other adult family members in this process, as well as your doctor. Drug testing, done under a doctor's supervision, may also help in the evaluation of your son for a substance abuse problem. If it turns out that he is abusing drugs, then further treatment is needed to help him get off the drugs, and stay away from them (see Table 12 for medications that are used in drug addiction). Useful links about substance abuse can be found under Question 100.

Table 12   Medications Used for the Treatment of Drug Addiction

Opiates
Buprenorphine
Naltrexone
Methadone, LAAM (long acting methadone)

Alcohol
Disulfiram
Naltrexone
Benzodiazepines
Anticonvulsants
Acamprosate
Ondansetron
Blood pressure medications
Typical and atypical antipsychotics

Cigarettes
Nicotine patch, gum, inhaler
Bupropion
Varenicline

Adapted from NIH Publication Number 07-5605: The Science Of Addiction.

40. My child has a learning disorder. Is that why he is depressed?

A learning disorder (e.g., math, reading, or other) per se is not usually the sole cause of a depression. However, the various difficulties associated with a learning disorder—constant frustration, embarrassment, or discouragement—can contribute negatively to a child's sense of accomplishment, his self-confidence, and feelings about himself among his peers. In a child who values academic achievement, a learning disability can create a tremendous amount of stress and demoralization. If a child struggles every day in school doing what his peers accomplish without much effort, he may generalize the way he feels about his failures in school into other areas of his life. He may feel he is a worthless person, and that he can't do anything right. He may adopt a negative outlook on everything. If this happens, depression could be the reaction of an unaddressed learning disorder. As the parent, what you may see could be constant irritability or low mood. The most useful way to address a learning disorder would be to seek the appropriate academic resources through school and other educators to help your child learn alternate ways to solve problems. Maybe your child needs additional services such as a resource room where specific subjects could be reviewed on an individual or semi-individual basis with another teacher or to be in a classroom environment that is different from the one in which he is currently enrolled. Sometimes a child with learning problems can benefit from having an **Individual Education Plan (IEP)**. An IEP is a written program that recommends what alternate or additional educational services a child should receive in school, normally unavailable to the majority of students. It may call for a smaller class size with a higher

---

Individual Education Plan (IEP)

This is a document created by educators for a child with special educational needs that may call for smaller class size, additional instruction in certain subjects such as math or reading, or additional services such as counseling and/or special therapies such as speech or handwriting (occupational therapy). Parental input is usually invited in the creation of an IEP.

teaching staff to child ratio in the room as compared to the general class environment, or it may indicate additional services such as a subject-specific resource room in reading or math, speech therapy, or other special therapies. The IEP is created by teachers and other educators and invites the parents' input. In New York City, the IEP is considered a document that classifies your child as receiving "Special Educational Services" ("Special Ed." in contrast to "General Ed."). Not all children with learning disabilities are classified as "Special Ed." for a variety of reasons. Some families do not want their children to be labeled as "different" or may feel their children will be perceived as "slow" by being classified. Other concerns may include worry that classification will hurt the child's future admission to the college of choice or other plans, since in some cases the high school diploma will look different. This is a discussion that is best had with your child's teacher or guidance counselor, who will have the experience needed to know if classification will benefit your child.

We often forget the impact a learning disorder in a child can have on the parents. For highly achieving parents, having a learning disordered child can be a huge blow to their own esteem. As parents, you can feel similar frustrations and disappointments as does your child over the academic hurdles. Your hopes for your child's future may seem compromised as a result of one or more learning problems. Sometimes a parent's worries with regard to the learning disability can surpass the child's. When this happens, it becomes yet another source of stress within the family. Though it may be difficult, try not to let your apprehension spill over too much in your interactions with your child. Your attitude sets the tone for how your child will feel about his problem; an anxious and negative attitude will be taken

We often forget the impact a learning disorder in a child can have on the parents.

up by your son as easily as a hopeful and optimistic one. Your doctor may be able to provide you with the support needed, or recommend someone else who could help navigate the difficulties of parenting a son who has both a mood disorder and a learning disorder.

41. If my child has more than one emotional problem at the same time, such as anxiety and depression, which should be treated first?

If a child has several emotional problems, the one which is causing the most distress and/or difficulty in functioning is generally treated first. Sometimes, treating the first one, such as disabling anxiety, can have the effect of alleviating the other. A healthcare provider may start an intensive course of psychotherapy with a child who is highly anxious and depressed and find that as the anxiety improves the depression is reduced as well. If medicines are needed, some of them, particularly the serotonin reuptake inhibitors (SSRIs), manage to treat symptoms of both depression and anxiety at the same time, so in such a case the two may not need to be separated at all (see Table 13 for medications used for anxiety).

You and your doctor can determine what the treatment priorities should be in the case of co-existing psychiatric disorders.

42. Why does my child cut herself?

Cutting is one example of many ways in which a child may cause harm to her body. Self-injurious behavior

Table 13 Medications Used to Treat Anxiety

Antidepressants
- Selective Serotonin Reuptake Inhibitors (SSRIs)
- Serotonin Noradrenergic Reuptake Inhibitors (SNRIs)—e.g., venlafaxine, duloxetine
- Tricyclic Antidepressants (TCAs)
- Monoamine Oxidase Inhibitors (MAOIs)

Benzodiazepines

Blood pressure medications (beta blockers, alpha agonists and antagonists)

Buspirone

Anticonvulsants

Atypical antipsychotics

includes inflicting deep or superficial lacerations of the skin using a sharp instrument like a knife, scratching with a needle, or inducing cuts in the skin with one's own nails. There are many other means to self-injure, some of which may appear more "benign" but nonetheless disfiguring such as obtaining tattoos or piercing different areas of the body. Sometimes self-injurious behavior is done secretly and the signs of it kept hidden from view, while at other times it is obvious. Why children, especially teenagers, engage in cutting or other self-injury is a difficult and complicated question. The teenager might want to make a statement to other people about how he is feeling. At times, the media—movies, television shows, books— may serve to glamorize or popularize cutting to a teenager. Teenagers may want to convey a social message by having certain marks on their bodies that identify with celebrities. Traditional cultures have sometimes used cutting the body for ritualistic and decorative purposes. Sometimes teens in our culture may cut themselves for those reasons as well—scars or tattoos can suggest gang affiliation, for example. Cutting may be something other than cosmetic for some teens. The act could represent aggression stemming from sadness or anger that is directed toward oneself. The act may provide some kind of relief from tension or frustration. Research has shown that cutting and inflicting pain causes the body to release chemicals in the blood that act as natural painkillers (**endogenous opiates**), and may even cause a low level of euphoria like that caused by a drug. Sometimes a teenager may think that he will be distracted and escape unpleasant feelings by cutting himself. People who cut may describe feeling a lot better after doing it. Occasionally, a youngster will cut himself as means to die, although usually he will not succeed in achieving that end. This situation is among the more serious motivations for cutting, and deserves immediate attention from a doctor.

Cutting is usually a symptom of some other underlying problem. For example, self-injurious behaviors occurring in the context of the low mood of major depressive episode may diminish or disappear completely as a person's symptoms of depression improve under treatment. Cutting may be a symptom of an emotional problem known as **Borderline Personality Disorder** (see Table 14), which can begin as a teenager and continue into adulthood. This disorder is characterized by self-injurious behavior, along with distortions in self-image, relationships with others, black and white thinking, fears of abandonment, and other features. As a parent, it's hard to see your child damage her own body in that way, and you will likely want to do anything you can to put a stop to it. While you may be upset by it, communicating your anger about it rarely helps reduce the behavior in your child, and may encourage it. You could express your concern about it,

Endogenous opiates

Naturally occurring chemicals in the body that are released by pain or stress, that result in numbing or decreased perception of pain.

Cutting is usually a symptom of some other underlying problem.

Borderline Personality Disorder

This disorder is characterized by self-injurious behavior, along with distortions in self-image, relationships with others, black and white thinking, fears of abandonment, and other features (see Table 14).

Table 14   Modified Criteria for Borderline Personality Disorder

A pervasive pattern of **instability of interpersonal relationships, self-image, and affects, and marked impulsivity** beginning by early adulthood and present in a variety of contexts, as indicated by **five (or more)** of the following:

- frantic efforts to avoid abandonment
- unstable and intense interpersonal relationships characterized by alternating between extremes of idealization and devaluation
- unstable self-image or sense of self
- impulsivity in at least two areas that are potentially self-damaging (e.g., spending, sex, substance abuse, reckless driving, binge eating)
- recurrent suicidality or self-injury
- marked reactivity of mood (e.g., intense episodic dysphoria, irritability, or anxiety usually lasting a few hours and only rarely more than a few days)
- chronic feelings of emptiness
- inappropriate, intense anger or difficulty controlling anger (e.g., frequent displays of temper, constant anger, recurrent physical fights)
- transient, stress-related paranoid thinking or dissociation

Note: Children and young adolescents are generally not diagnosed with this disorder, although features of the disorder may be seen in this population.

(Adapted with permission from the *Diagnostic and Statistical Manual of Mental Disorders*, Text Revision, Fourth Edition. Copyright 2000. American Psychiatric Association.)

however. If you can get your teenager to talk about it, that's an important first step. Adolescents usually will not be able to answer the question of "why" they are cutting, but maybe what they are feeling when they do it. Your doctor may be able to help foster a discussion about it, and have recommendations on how to treat the behaviors further. Specific treatments for cutting behaviors in patients with Borderline Personality Disorder are available, which include certain types of psychotherapy, and possibly medications. Your child's doctor will be able to recommend the most appropriate treatment or make a referral to someone who can provide it.

Diagnosis

73

43. My family is from another country. Isn't depression a "Western" problem?

Many cultures do not view depression or mental illness in the same way as we do in the United States. It may not be seen as problem that is separate from the body. For example, some Asian cultures see depression as an imbalance within the body which needs correction by performing certain actions or taking certain preparations such as herbs or homeopathic products. It may be a source of embarrassment or shame, and because of that, its existence may be denied altogether. In some cultures, the stigma of mental illness in an individual can bring social compromise to an entire family, encouraging the afflicted person (or his parent) to be shunned or even punished. Some cultures have a religious explanation for why a mental illness occurred, and that restoration of faith or performing religious rituals should improve the symptoms.

No matter what country of origin or culture, studies from various communities around the world show that depression and bipolar disorder are not unique to Western society. Seeking help can be the first step in overcoming the problem. Bringing cultural issues into the treatment is an important part of treatment and recovery. Sometimes, families from another culture will avoid psychiatric treatment because they feel that they will not be understood, or that they will be humiliated in the eyes of the dominant culture. On the other hand, other cultures often have strengths which can be used to help in the recovery, once the psychiatric problem is identified. You may be able to teach your doctor about your culture, and help her come to an understanding of your special concerns, so that they can be integrated into a **treatment plan** that will work well for you and your family.

44. Our 12-year-old nephew was recently diagnosed with diabetes and needs to take insulin. Since this happened, he has been sad all the time. Can it be depression?

Your nephew may be experiencing depression, although it may be too soon to say if it is a full MDE. It is not uncommon for anyone, adult or child, to experience a strong reaction to the diagnosis of a major medical condition. The reaction may include feelings anger or sadness at being "different" from other children. Alternatively, as with a death or loss, the reaction may be a bereavement process at losing one's health or innocence. Major lifestyle changes such as diet, frequent and painful finger sticks to monitor blood sugar, and the administration of insulin by needles, can all cause emotional distress in a newly diagnosed diabetic patient. Symptoms such as sadness, irritability, anxiety, poor appetite/sleep/concentration, may be seen in such a case. An adjustment disorder with a depressed or anxious mood or an MDE may be diagnosed. However, it is important to involve a doctor and other professionals in evaluating such symptoms in your nephew. Often, a number of health professionals, such as a nurse or social worker, as well as doctors, may be involved in the evaluation and care of a diabetic child. If this team of professionals feels that your nephew's reactions are in need of further attention from a mental health standpoint, they will usually indicate this to

Treatment plan

A written document in the medical record or a conceptual outline used by the clinician that names important goals in a child's psychiatric treatment.

Diagnosis

the family, and may have resources readily available for this purpose.

In addition to different treatments for emotional distress ranging from informal counseling by the medical team, to more involved individual and family therapy conducted by mental health professionals, those with medical conditions such as diabetes often benefit from group treatment. This may include family education or support groups, as well as groups for children who have the illness in common to help them learn to cope with the challenges of that illness.

PART FOUR

Treatment

What are the usual treatments available for
childhood mood disorders?

What medications are used to treat childhood
depression and bipolar disorder?

How do psychiatric medications affect my child's
growth and development?

I don't believe in traditional medicines. Are there
alternative treatments that I can give my
depressed child?

More . . .

45. What are the usual treatments available for childhood mood disorders?

A number of treatments exist and are typically used for mood disorders. These include many types of individual psychotherapy (known as "talk therapy" in lay terms), family and group psychotherapy, medications, and psychoeducation (patient and family education using discussion or literature—written or electronic—on various topics relevant to psychiatric issues), as well as assistance with academic and social functioning. Parent training, where parents are taught how to interact with their children and manage difficult behavior in a more productive manner, is also a treatment option that may be used to complement other treatments already employed.

Often, the treatments described here will be accessed through an individual mental health professional privately or in a clinic setting usually one to two times a week or perhaps once a month. This means of receiving treatment is called treatment in an ambulatory or outpatient setting. For more severely impaired children, ambulatory treatment may require a more intensive level of service such as that available in a day hospital or day treatment program. These programs provide more psychiatric supervision, usually on a daily basis, and are considered a step down from hospitalization. Sometimes additional services may be available through social service agencies for families in ambulatory treatment. These services include the assignment of trained workers (case managers) who meet with the family in their homes and in the community to help with parenting skills, crisis management, and other treatment issues. A hospital environment is usually reserved for short-term management of the most extreme or dangerous behaviors exhibited by a child, with the goal of returning back home when he is more stable. Occasionally, children unable to be treated successfully while living at home do better in highly structured and controlled environments such as hospitals. Under these circumstances, these children might be considered for treatment by living in a supervised residence with other such children. Different levels of structure and supervision exist within residential settings, depending on the needs of the child. The AACAP Facts for Families series has a more detailed information sheet, entitled, "The Continuum of Care for Children and Families" which further explains some of these different treatment options (see Question 100 for details).

46. How does one decide whether to use medicine or psychotherapy in treating depression or BPD?

Every case is different, and no one approach to treatment is considered the standard for all children and adolescents with mood disorders. Some patients may do well, especially those with mild to moderate depression, or an adjustment disorder, with only psychotherapy. Yet others, such as those with BPD, severe depression, or comorbid conditions, will need medications to complement other treatments to recover. If family members with the same illness have had positive response to certain medications, often those medicines receive strong consideration in the child's treatment. A combination of medicine, psychotherapy, and other approaches that incorporate school and social functioning may be needed to treat a pediatric mood disorder. Your doctor should be able to discuss the options with you in further detail, and help determine which treatments are most appropriate.

47. What did my doctor mean when he said he would be using "psychotropic" medications to treat my son?

Psychotropic medications refer to medicines that specifically affect the brain. They include antidepressants, mood stabilizers including antiseizure medications, antipsychotics, stimulants, and other medicines that have use with psychiatric disorders. This term is used in contrast to other medications children may receive such as those used for asthma or stomach disorders, which usually have little effect on the brain, and have no specific role in treating emotions or behavior.

Psychotropic medications

Medications which act specifically and primarily upon the brain, in contrast to other parts of the body, as in the case of asthma medications acting upon the lungs (but not the brain).

48. What medications are used to treat childhood depression and bipolar disorder?

Depression is usually treated with antidepressants (see Tables 15–17). These include the selective serotonin reuptake inhibitors (SSRIs), the tricyclic antidepressants (TCAs), the monoamine oxidase inhibitors (MAOIs), and several others categories of antidepressants, as well as with mood stabilizers and antipsychotics (see Table 18). In cases of comorbid disorders such as ADHD, other agents normally used to control inattentive, impulsive, or hyperactive symptoms such as the stimulants or blood pressure medications may also be used (see Table 10). You may be unfamiliar

Table 15 Tricyclic Antidepressants and Monoamine Oxidase Inhibitors

TCAs

clomipramine (Anafranil)

amitriptyline (Elavil)

doxepin (Sinequan)

trimipramine (Surmontil)

amoxapine (Asendin)

protriptyline (Vivactil)

desipramine (Norpramin)

nortriptyline (Pamelor, Aventyl)

imipramine (Tofranil, Tofranil-PM)

maprotiline (Ludiomil)

MAOIs

phenelzine (Nardil)

tranylcypromine (Parnate)

with the generic names of medicines, but instead may recognize certain brand names from among these medicines. With all the information available from the pharmaceutical industry and the Internet about different medications, it can be very confusing at times. As a patient or family member of a patient, you would not need to decide what medicine you want to use in treatment, since your psychiatrist will generally offer you recommendations based on your child's presentation. However, your consent will be needed to start the medication, and your participation in the form of frequent communication is essential to monitor the response to the treatment. Tables 15–18 indicate the variety of choices available in treatment, and may be helpful for families to get a sense of the options that their doctor is choosing in the treatment.

Bipolar disorder may be treated with any of the mentioned categories of antidepressants during the depressed

Table 16 Selective Serotonin Reuptake Inhibitors (SSRIs)

Generic Name	Brand Name	How Supplied	Dosage Range/ Frequency
Citalopram	Celexa	10 mg, 20 mg, 40 mg tab	10–40 mg/day given once a day
	Celexa oral solution	2 mg/mL	
Escitalopram	Lexapro	5 mg, 10 mg, 20 mg	10–20 mg/day given once a day
	Lexapro oral solution	1 mg/mL	
Fluoxetine	Prozac,	10 mg, 20 mg, 40 mg Pulvules	10–60 mg/day given once a day
	Sarafem	10 mg, 20 mg, 40 mg capsules	10–60 mg/day given once a day
		10 mg tab	10–60 mg/day given once a day
	Prozac oral solution	20 mg/5 mL	10–60 mg/day given once a day
	Prozac weekly delayed release	90 mg capsule	90 mg given once a week
Fluvoxamine	Luvox	25 mg, 50 mg, 100 mg tab	100–300 mg given once a day
	Luvox CR (extended release)	100 mg, 150 mg capsules	
Paroxetine	Paxil	10 mg, 20 mg, 30 mg, 40 mg tab	10–50 mg/day given once a day
	Paxil oral suspension	10 mg/5 mL	
	Paxil CR controlled release	12.5 mg, 25 mg, 37.5 mg tab	12.5–62.5 mg/day given once a day
Sertraline	Zoloft	25 mg, 50 mg, 100 mg tab	25–200 mg/day given once a day
	Zoloft oral concentrate	20 mg/mL	Given once a day

Prophylaxis

The use of medication to prevent the occurrence of an episode of illness.

Anticonvulsants

Medications used to treat or prevent seizures. This family of medications often has utility in the treatment of BPD for mood stabilization (see Table 18).

Antipsychotics

Medications used to treat psychosis (hallucinations, delusions, or other distortions in the perception of reality).

or mixed phase of the illness, but precautions are needed to avoid the possibility of inducing mania. During the manic or mixed phase of BPD, and for **prophylaxis** against manic episodes, mood stabilizers such as lithium, **anticonvulsants**, and/or **antipsychotics** are generally used.

Table 17   Other Antidepressants

Generic Name	Brand Name	How Supplied	Dosage Range/ Frequency
Buproprion	Wellbutrin	75 mg, 100 mg tab	100–450 mg/day given in divided doses 2–3 times/day
	Wellbutrin SR	100 mg, 150 mg, 200 mg tab	100–450 mg/day given in divided doses 2 times/day
	Zyban (sustained release)	150 mg tab	150–300 mg/day given in divided doses 2 times/day
	Wellbutrin XL	150 mg, 300 mg tab	150–450 mg/day given once a day
Duloxetine (delayed release)	Cymbalta	20 mg, 30 mg, 60 mg capsules	20–60 mg/day given in divided doses 1–2 times/day
Mirtazapine	Remeron	15 mg, 30 mg, 45 mg tab	15–45 mg/day given once a day
Nefazodone	Serzone	50 mg, 100 mg, 150 mg, 200 mg, 250 mg tab	100–600 mg/day given in divided doses 2 times a day
Trazodone	Desyrel	50 mg, 100 mg, 150 mg, 300 mg	100–400 mg/day given once at bedtime
Venlafaxine	Effexor	25 mg, 37.5 mg, 50 mg, 75 mg, 100 mg	75–375 mg/day given in divided doses 2 times a day
	Effexor XR (extended release)	37.5 mg, 75 mg, 150 mg	75–225 mg/day, given once a day

49. What is "off label use" of medication?

Prescribing medications that are not approved by the United States Food and Drug Administration (FDA) for a particular illness in a specific population is called "off label use." The FDA approves a drug only after a substantial amount of patient research has been done to support its safety and benefits. It takes many years to collect the necessary information from research to gain FDA approval for a medication. The FDA will

Table 18   Mood Stabilizing Medications

Generic Name	Brand Name	How Supplied	Dosage Range/ Frequency
Lithium*			*150–1800 mg/day*
Lithium carbonate	Eskalith	150 mg, 300 mg tablets or capsules	Divided into 2–3 doses/day
Lithium carbonate, slow release (extended release)	Lithobid	300 mg tablets	Divided into 2 doses/day
	Eskalith-CR	450 mg tablets	Divided into 2 doses/day
Lithium citrate	Cibalith-S syrup	syrup 8 mEq/ 5 mL (300 mg of lithium/5 mL)	Divided into 2–3 doses/day
Anticonvulsants			
Carbema-zepine*	Tegretol	100 mg, 200 mg tab	100–1600 mg/day
	Tegretol syrup	100 mg/5 mL syrup	Divided into 2–4 doses/day
	Tegretol	100 mg chewable tab	Divided into 2–4 doses/day
	Tegretol-XR (extended release)	100 mg, 200 mg, 400 mg tab	Divided into 2 doses/day
	Carbatrol (extended release)	100 mg, 200 mg, 300 mg tab	Divided into 2 doses/day
Divalproex sodium* (enteric coated)	Depakote	125 mg, 250 mg, 500 mg tab	250–2000 mg/day divided 2–3 doses/day
	Depakote ER	250 mg, 500 mg tab	Divided 1–2 doses/day
	Depakote	125 mg capsule (sprinkle)	Divided 2–3 doses/day
Gabapentin	Neurontin, Gabapentin	100 mg, 300 mg, 400 mg cap/tab 600mg, 800mg tab	300–2000 mg/day divided into 2–3 doses/day
	Neurontin syrup	250 mg/5mL	Divided into 2–3 doses/day
Lamotrigine	Lamictal	25 mg, 100 mg, 150 mg, 200 mg tab	25–400mg/day divided into 1–2 doses/day
	Lamictal chewable	2 mg, 5 mg, 25 mg tab	Divided into 1–2 doses/day

(Continued next page)

Table 18   (continued)

Generic Name	Brand Name	How Supplied	Dosage Range/ Frequency
Levetiracetam	Keppra	250 mg, 500 mg, 750 mg tab	500–3000 mg/day divided into 2 doses/day
	Keppra XR	500 mg, 750 mg, 1000 mg	Once a day
	Keppra syrup	100 mg/mL	Divided into 2 doses/day
Oxcarbemazepine	Trileptal	150 mg, 300 mg, 600 mg	600–2400 mg/day divided into 2 doses/day
	Trileptal syrup	300 mg/5mL	Divided into 2 doses/day
Topiramate	Topamax	25 mg, 50 mg, 100 mg, 200 mg tab	25–400 mg/day divided into 2 doses/day
	Topamax	15 mg, 25 mg cap (sprinkle)	Divided into 2 doses/day
Tiagabine	Gabitril	2 mg, 4 mg, 12 mg, 16 mg, 20 mg tab	4–56mg/day Divided into 2–4 doses/day
Valproic acid*	Depakene	250 mg cap	250–2000 mg/day divided into 2–3 doses/day
	Depakene syrup	250 mg/5mL	Divided into 2–3 doses/day
Zonisamide	Zonegran	25 mg, 50 mg, 100 mg cap	100–600 mg/day divided into 1–2 doses/day

Atypical Antipsychotics

Arapiprazole	Abilify	2 mg, 5 mg, 10 mg, 15 mg, 20 mg, 30 mg tab	2.5–30 mg/day once a day
	Abilify Discmelt (rapid dissolving)	10 mg, 15 mg tab	Once a day
	Abilify oral solution	1 mg/mL	Once a day
	Abilify injection	9.75 mg/1.3 mL dose	Once a day
Clozapine*	Clozaril,	25 mg, 100 mg tab	12.5–900 mg/day divided into 1–2 doses/day
	FazaClo (rapid dissolving)	12.5 mg, 25 mg, 100 mg	1–2 doses/day

(Continued next page)

85

Table 18   (continued)

Generic Name	Brand Name	How Supplied	Dosage Range/ Frequency
Olanzapine	Zyprexa	2.5 mg, 5 mg, 7.5 mg, 10 mg, 15 mg, 20 mg tab	2.5–30 mg/day once a day
Zyprexa	Zyprexa, Zydis (rapid dissolving)	5 mg, 10 mg, 15 mg, 20 mg tab	Once a day
Quetiapine	Seroquel	25 mg, 50 mg, 100 mg, 200 mg, 300 mg, 400 mg tab	100–800mg/day divided into 2 doses/day
	Seroquel XR (extended release)	50 mg, 150 mg, 200 mg, 300 mg, 400 mg tab	Once a day
Risperidone	Risperdal	0.5 mg, 1 mg, 2 mg, 3 mg, 4 mg tab	1–2 doses/day, 0.5–4 mg/day
	Risperdal M-tab (rapid dissolving)	0.25 mg, 0.5 mg, 1 mg, 2 mg, 3 mg, 4 mg tab	1–2 doses/day
	Risperdal Consta	12.5 mg, 25 mg, 37.5 mg, 50 mg/vial	1 dose injected/2 weeks (injectable, long acting)
Ziprasidone	Geodon	20 mg, 40 mg, 60 mg, 80 mg capsules	80–200 mg/day divided into 2 doses a day
	Geodon	20 mg/vial	Emergency use every 2–4 hours (injectable)

*Periodic blood levels are required.

not approve a drug for children unless the research is done specifically using pediatric populations. For a variety of reasons, research in children and adolescents is considerably more limited than those in adults, but it is slowly increasing. Relatively few psychiatric medications have received FDA approval for use in children, aside from those used for ADHD (for which there are many approved medicines). These include fluoxetine for depression, lithium for mania, a few medicines for obsessive compulsive disorder, bedwetting, psychosis, and **Tourette's disorder**. This leaves dozens of other

Tourette's disorder
A childhood onset disorder characterized by motor and vocal tics. Tics are a type of sudden, repetitive movements or vocal sounds.

psychotropic medicines, while approved for adults, available to children only in a manner that is considered "off label." The serious consequences of untreated psychiatric illness in children and adolescents lead a large number of psychiatrists to consider "off label" use of medications in their patients, in addition to other therapeutic options. "Off label" use in the professional community is done often, and widely accepted as long as the doctor feels the medicine is appropriate for the child's particular condition, the medication is carefully monitored, and used in a cautious manner. Finally, "off label" use of medications in child and adolescent psychiatry encourages further research in the use of these medicines and possibly future approval by the FDA.

50. What are the common side effects seen with medications for mood disorders?

Side effects experienced during the treatment of mood disorders depend on the type of medication used. Most side effects are not dangerous, but rather bothersome. Less often, a side effect could be more serious, and may be a reason to monitor the medicine more closely or stop the medicine altogether. Side effects are frequently worse in the beginning of treatment with a new medication and may improve as the body gets used to having the medication in its system. Occasionally, some side effects continue indefinitely, and the challenge in taking the medicine will be to balance the benefits over the inconveniences. Just of few of the types of medication side effects are mentioned here, as the full list is rather extensive. The package insert or pharmacy information sheet will generally present you with an exhaustive list of potential side effects. In any case, a more thorough discussion with your doctor is helpful

The serious consequences of untreated psychiatric illness in children and adolescents lead a large number of psychiatrists to consider "off label" use of medications in their patients, in addition to other therapeutic options.

Treatment

to anticipate possible side effects of your child's own medication regimen.

Side effects for SSRIs and other antidepressants may include sedation or wakefulness, an inner feeling of restlessness, weight gain, constipation or stomach upset, or dry mouth. A more serious side effect of the SSRIs and other antidepressants that will be further discussed in Question 56 is the possible increase in suicidality at the beginning of treatment (see Table 19). Lithium can cause acne, weight gain, sedation, increased urination, or problems with the thyroid or kidney functioning. Other mood stabilizers such as valproic acid can cause weight gain, sedation, or interfere with the body's ability to make enough blood cells or other components of the blood (see Table 20). The antipsychotic medications (see Table 21) can cause weight gain, sedation, dry mouth, dizziness, blurred vision, or constipation. More serious side effects of antipsychotic medication, further discussed in the response to Question 64, include diabetes, the development of an irreversible, abnormal movement disorder (**tardive dyskinesia**), or an illness that includes high fever and stiffness of the muscles (**neuroleptic malignant syndrome**). Several of the medications described can cause slowed thinking or memory problems.

Tardive dyskinesia

A permanent movement disorder that may occur months to years after using antipsychotic medications.

Neuroleptic malignant syndrome

Known commonly as "NMS." This is a life-threatening, but rare condition brought on by antipsychotic use.

51. How do psychiatric medications affect my child's growth and development?

The impact of psychiatric medications on a child's general growth and development is not fully known. This is partly because long term studies comparing growth and development with children who are on and off medicines are ongoing and incomplete. Also, many

Table 19   Adverse Effects of Antidepressants by Class*

Medication class	Potential Adverse Effects
SSRIs	nausea, diarrhea, insomnia, anxiety, nervousness, dizziness, somnolence, tremor, decreased libido, sweating, anorexia, dry mouth, headache, sexual dysfunction, **serotonin syndrome**
TCAs	dry mouth, constipation, nausea, anorexia, weight gain, sweating, increased appetite, nervousness, decreased libido, dizziness, tremor, somnolence, blurred vision, tachycardia, urinary hesitancy, hypotension, cardiac toxicity
MAOIs	dizziness, headache, drowsiness, hypotension, insomnia, agitation, dry mouth, constipation, nausea, urinary hesitancy, weight gain, edema, sexual dysfunction, increased liver enzymes, toxic food and drug interactions

Others (drugs listed separately)

bupropion (Wellbutrin)	weight loss, dry mouth, rash, sweating, agitation, dizziness, insomnia, nausea, abdominal pain, weakness, headache, blurred vision, constipation, tremor, rapid heart rate, ringing in ears, seizures
venlafaxine (Effexor)	sweating, nausea, constipation, decreased appetite, vomiting, insomnia, somnolence, dry mouth, dizziness, nervousness, tremor, blurred vision, sexual dysfunction, rapid heart rate, hypertension
duloxetine (Cymbalta)	nausea, dry mouth, constipation, loss of appetite, fatigue, drowsiness, dizziness, sweating, blurred vision, rash, itching, sexual dysfunction, tremor, unusual bleeding
mirtazapine (Remeron)	somnolence, appetite increase, weight gain, dizziness, dry mouth, constipation, hypotension, abnormal dreams, flu syndrome, low blood cell counts
nefazodone (Serzone)	somnolence, dry mouth, nausea, dizziness, insomnia, agitation, constipation, abnormal vision, confusion, liver failure
trazodone (Desyrel)	sedation, hypotension, dizziness, blurred vision, headache, loss of appetite, sweating, restlessness, rapid heart rate, prolonged erection

*Listed adverse effects are not exhaustive of side effects as reported in the *Physicians' Desk Reference*. Rather more common effects within each group were included, as well as some more serious effects. Side effect profiles of medications within a class may vary. Any concern about an adverse effect from a medication should be discussed with your doctor.

Serotonin Syndrome

A situation created by taking an excess of medications that boosts serotonin activity in the body. It includes sweating, tremor, agitation, various neurologic symptoms like increased muscle reactivity and mental confusion.

Treatment

Table 20   Adverse Effects of Selected Mood Stabilizers

Name	Common Side Effects	More Serious Side Effects
Lithium (Eskalith, Lithobid)	Acne, increased thirst and urination, tremor, hair loss, stomach upset, diarrhea, kidney changes and reduced kidney function, thyroid toxicity, weight gain, benign increase in white blood cell count, dermatitis and other skin reactions	Neurologic and cardiac toxicity in overdose
Valproic acid/ divalproex sodium (Depakene/ Depakote)	Stomach upset, diarrhea, hair loss, weight gain, low platelet count/ bruising or bleeding, tremor, imbalance and coordination problems, sedation	Liver failure, neurologic toxicity, severe drug rash
Carbemazepine (Tegretol, Carbatrol)	Sedation, low white blood cell count, slurred speech, coordination problems, imbalance, stomach upset, double and blurred vision, thinking and memory problems	Severe drug rash, dangerously low white blood cell count, suppression of red blood cell and platelet production
Lamotrigine (Lamictal)	Stomach upset, visual problems, imbalance	Severe, potentially fatal drug rash
Topiramate (Topamax)	Dizziness, numbness and tingling, sedation, nausea, loss of appetite, confusion, concentration problems	Severe metabolic acidosis

studies about the effect of medications on the brain are done in adult populations, so the child equivalents are not known. What's more, psychotropic medications used in adults may have no effect on some types of growth and development which are still occurring in children. An example of a child-specific concern with medication is illustrated by the controversy raised about the effect on a child's height of psychostimulants, a type of medication used to treat ADHD. Research done over the last 30–40 years has shown that these medications may cause children on treat-

Table 21   Adverse Effects of Atypical Antipsychotics

Generic Name	Brand Name	Common Side Effects	More Serious Effects
Clozapine	Clozaril, FazaClo	Constipation, sedation, akathisia, increased salivation, weight gain, increased heart rate, dry mouth	Agranulocytosis (failure to produce white blood cells), neuroleptic malignant syndrome (NMS), tardive dyskinesia (TD), diabetes, future cardiometabolic risks
Aripiprazole	Abilify	Constipation, akathisia, possible weight gain, constipation, blurred vision, muscle stiffness	NMS, TD, diabetes, future cardiometabolic risks
Risperidone	Risperdal	Constipation, akathisia, weight gain, abnormal lactation, blurred vision, muscle stiffness	NMS, TD, diabetes, future cardiometabolic risks
Olanzapine	Zyprexa	Constipation, akathesia, weight gain, blurred vision, muscle stiffness	NMS, TD, diabetes, future cardiometabolic risks
Ziprasidone	Geodon	Constipation, akathesia, possible weight gain, muscle stiffness	NMS, TD, diabetes, future cardiometabolic risks, cardiac toxicity

ment to grow more slowly than those who are not on treatment. However, more recent studies have shown that many children on such medications have periods of "catch up growth" when given "medication holidays" (periods of time such as weekends or vacations where medicine is not given at all) and have achieved similar heights by the time they reach adulthood as those of their non-medicated peers. Researchers also have wondered if children with ADHD have a different growth pattern than those without, and if that reflects some of these results as well. Adults with ADHD do not need to concern themselves with this issue of height and psychostimulants, whereas parents of a short child with ADHD may have hesitations about this class of medication.

The long term effects of certain medicines on children often remains unclear. Many parents are especially concerned about the effects of psychotropic medications on a child's brain development. This is certainly a legitimate concern since medications do change the way neurons function while the child is taking those medicines and may ultimately direct how different areas of the brain operate, not only in childhood but at any age. In some cases, research has shown that adult brains of people with certain psychiatric disorders can show positive changes in structure and/or function as seen on **neuroimaging tests** (pictures of the brain) after treatment with medications. The damaging effects on the adult brain from illegal drugs has been shown using these types of tests as well (this is certainly part of the reason why they're illegal). Animal studies have shown that stress and traumatic events can have negative effects on the structure and function of the brain. Some research suggests that psychotropic medications could have a reparative or protective effect on the brains of those who are predisposed to psychiatric illness. For these individuals, treatment with medications may offer a more positive direction for growth and development to occur. The many questions about the impact of psychotropic medications on the brain lead psychiatrists to be both more conservative at times in their use of psychotropic medications, and more liberal, as compared to their use in adults. Some doctors feel the benefits of psychotropic medicines are outweighed by the long-term uncertainties about the effect on growth (the more conservative group), where others feel that the risks of under-treating child psychiatric illness and chances of long term disabilities in

Many parents are especially concerned about the effects of psychotropic medications on a child's brain development.

Neuroimaging tests

Commonly known as "brain scans," these include computer tomography (CT or CAT scans), magnetic resonance imaging (MRIs), and other tests looking at the structure of the brain or its function.

personal, social and academic functioning far outweigh these uncertainties (the more liberal group).

52. How did our doctor decide which medicine is the best one for our daughter's depression? There are so many out there and they all sound alike!

Doctors make decisions about medications based on their own experience, professional guidelines, and available research. The best way to clarify how a choice of medication was made is to have a discussion with your doctor. Child psychiatrists tend to use the SSRIs more often than the older types of antidepressant medicines such as the TCAs or MAOIs due to the lower risk of overdose or interaction with another drug or food. Some of the medicines have side effects that affect sleep or appetite. Careful choice of such medicines can help a child's symptoms of illness, rather than worsen them. Some psychotropic medications come in liquid, rapid dissolving, or extremely low dose tablet forms. These may be desirable when younger children or very sensitive children are being treated. Many medications are now available in once-a-day, long acting forms, which can be more convenient than medicines administered two to four times a day. If a child has a seizure disorder as well as a mood disorder, an anticonvulsant or a combination of anticonvulsants may be chosen for mood stabilization over another agent like lithium. Some medications require periodic blood tests to check drug levels in the body or other monitoring tests to check the effects of the medicine on the body. Such medicines may be less desirable for a child who has an aversion to getting blood drawn, over one where infrequent monitoring is required.

In summary, the factors that influence the choice of medication for depression or any other mood disorder include safety and side effect profiles, ease of administration/dosing, utility in other comorbid conditions, and monitoring requirements. More specific questions, such as why one antidepressant or mood stabilizer was chosen over another in the same class, are best directed to your doctor, who can explain why the choice was made.

53. How can we manage weight gain with medications used to treat our daughter's mood disorder?

Weight gain and being overweight are among the biggest challenges faced today, not only by families with children who have emotional disorders, but also among healthy children in the pediatric community.

Weight gain and being overweight are among the biggest challenges faced today, not only by families with children who have emotional disorders, but also among healthy children in the pediatric community. In the United States, obesity among children and adolescents is felt to occur at unbelievably high rates. What's more, many of our primary care doctors feel helpless in the obesity crisis due to lack of time and resources.

The reasons for this epidemic of obesity are thought to be numerous. Some of these include the popularity through marketing of "fast foods" and other "junk foods" (which are high in fat and calories but low in nutrition), the limited opportunities for children to engage in physical activities in school and in the community, and the sedentary lifestyle that is furthered by society's dependence on the computer, television, or other electronic equipment. Genetics also plays a role in determining who becomes overweight and who does not, but since that is not a controllable factor, diet and lifestyle are the factors that are usually emphasized in weight management.

As if the tendency for children to gain weight in our society were not enough, weight management for children with psychiatric problems is often further complicated by the frequent side effect of weight gain from their psychotropic medications. This unfortunate reality can have a serious impact on your child's self-esteem as well as future health. It may argue against using certain medicines in your child if the weight gain exceeds the benefits of alleviating mood symptoms. Or, if the benefits of the medicine are slow to appear, this unwanted side effect may pose an argument to discontinue the medication. Before making any decisions about whether to stop a medication or pursue other means of losing weight, you are encouraged to discuss the problem with your child's doctor. You and your doctor may determine that every strategy available for weight loss needs to be implemented. These include consultation with your pediatrician, a nutritional evaluation (if available), a diet and exercise plan specific to weight reduction in children and adolescents, and other options such as a change in the medication regimen or addition of a different medicine. Parents will often describe the challenge of putting a child on a diet. Frequently, the whole family needs to be on a diet in order for the overweight child to successfully lose weight. A family diet plan would require that the home be stocked with healthy food, that junk food be reduced or eliminated from the cabinets and refrigerator, and that the family make a commitment to eat out less and cook more. Families are also encouraged to exercise together as a way of helping children lose weight. Teenagers could be harder or easier to engage in weight loss planning than younger children. It's especially helpful if your community has special group programs aimed at weight reduction and management available to teenagers.

An important feature of successful weight loss is that both the individual and family members have the motivation to make the necessary changes. If a child is discouraged or disinterested in keeping to a diet or participating in physical activities as part of a plan to lose weight but the parent is motivated, it can create yet another source of conflict and tension within the family. If you're ready to pursue a weight loss plan but your child isn't, you might discuss it in the treatment and consider ways to encourage your child further toward that goal. The National Heart, Lung, and Blood Institute (NHLBI) offers helpful tips on weight management at their "We Can!" website, and an example of a diet diary is provided, both noted in Question 100.

Geraldine's comment:
Both my kids make poor food choices. Lexie especially craves carbohydrates and they would rather have sugar over protein any day. Right now, their weights are good, but since we're venturing into some of the "big guns" in treatment like a trial on an SSRI for Lexie, we have to be aware of our eating habits, and the risk of huge weight gain. It's not easy once they're in middle school and the parent has less and less control of their diets.

54. What are SSRIs and how do they work in children?

The selective serotonin reuptake inhibitors (SSRIs) are a class of antidepressant medications that cause the neurotransmitter, serotonin, to remain between nerve cells in the brain and other parts of the body for a longer period of time than what naturally occurs. Serotonin is associated with feeling happy, calm, and a host of other functions in the nervous system. Serotonin is normally broken down or taken up from the spaces between nerve cells after a brief period of time. One theory of depression suggests that the amount of neurotransmitters such as serotonin and norepinephrine in the spaces between cells are in short supply. By blocking a protein in the part of the nerve cell before the space, the SSRI allows serotonin to remain in place longer and in increased amounts, causing an improvement in mood and alleviation of anxiety. Serotonin's effect on the body depends on the actions of the serotonin **receptor** (a special protein on the receiving end of a nerve cell) into which the serotonin fits. More than 10 types of serotonin receptors have been identified. Changes in the number of serotonin receptors and sensitivity of these receptors to serotonin occur with SSRI treatment over several weeks, also resulting in improved mood and reduced anxiety. The length of time needed for these changes to take place may explain why a full **response** to treatment with SSRIs is frequently not seen for 2–3 months.

Many SSRIs are available on the market (see Table 16). Each one is not necessarily equivalent to the other—some are more sedating, some last longer in the body or are metabolized more quickly. Choices are made according to the needs of the patient. If a response to the first SSRI is not seen, the psychiatrist may switch over to another category of antidepressant (see Question 56 for more information) or may try a different SSRI. Alternatively, an SSRI that is considered to be ineffective or only partially effective may be augmented (see Question 60 on augmentation) with another medication to help boost the effects.

Receptor

A structure on the end of a receiving nerve cell into which a traveling neurotransmitter such as serotonin can attach. Once a neurotransmitter has attached to a receptor, further changes in the chemical activity of the cell may occur. Different chemical activities among antidepressants as well as the side effects experienced are often defined by the receptors that they act upon.

Response

Reduction or resolution of psychiatric symptoms. A partial response to treatment during a depressive or manic episode is a reduced number of symptom criteria, while a full response results in a complete resolution of symptoms (also known as remission).

Treatment

55. What is the "black box warning" associated with antidepressants?

The United States government monitors and evaluates medications through the Food and Drug Administration (FDA). Drug manufacturers are required to provide detailed information about their products to patients and doctors, including side effects and warnings about risks as well as benefits. According to the FDA, the "black box" warning is the most serious type of warning that can be placed in the packaging of a medication. In 2004, the FDA concluded that the "black box" warning should be placed on product information for all SSRI and other antidepressants because their review of important patient research on more than 4,000 children and adolescents showed an increase in suicidal thoughts and suicidal behaviors (suicidality) in the early phase of treatment with these medicines. The recommendation has since been expanded to include a risk for suicidality in young adults up to age 25 as well. None of the people in the studies actually committed suicide but, because of the apparent increase in suicidality (4% in patients treated with antidepressants vs. 2% in patients treated with a **placebo**) the FDA wanted the highest level of warning and supervision for such medications. Recommendations were also made for a closer level of monitoring when first prescribing these medicines which ask that the doctor see the child more frequently for the first 3 months of treatment, when risks may be highest.

Since the issuance of the "black box" warning on SSRIs, the FDA has asked for a closer look at the original research used to draw conclusions about increased suicidality. Experts in the field of suicide, including Dr. Kelly Posner and others at the Columbia University/

Drug manufacturers are required to provide detailed information about their products to patients and doctors, including side effects and warnings about risks as well as benefits.

Placebo

A pill used in research which resembles the study drug, but is actually a "dummy" or "sugar" pill that contains no active drug.

New York State Psychiatric Institute were commissioned by the FDA to further analyze suicidality in the previous studies using a special questionnaire. The newer study revealed that suicidality was interpreted differently by doctors and others doing the original research. It also showed that less suicide attempts occurred than what was originally concluded. What did these newer studies accomplish for FDA approval process and real-life situations with doctors and patients? The FDA now requires drug companies to conduct special suicide assessments using the questionnaire developed by Dr. Posner and colleagues to ensure consistent evaluation of suicidality between different researchers. The newer studies have also created a greater awareness among doctors using antidepressant medications to conduct careful and thorough suicide evaluations of their patients on treatment.

The "black box" warning may be frightening to you, and with good reason. A parent could never forgive herself if she encouraged her child to take a medicine that would lead to suicide. However, bear in mind that untreated depression, bipolar, or other psychiatric disorders can also lead to suicide. That would also be hard to forgive. The connection between suicidal behavior and medication versus suicide and depression itself is hard to distinguish. Many depressed young people, treated with medications or not, have suicidal thoughts and make attempts on their lives. The 1999 U.S Surgeon General's report noted that more than 500,000 young people in this country attempt suicide and about 2,000 of them succeed. The same report also stated that the rates of suicide among youth are decreasing as compared to previous years. This decrease is frequently attributed to the improved treatments for depression and other psychiatric disorders,

Treatment

Newer studies have created a greater awareness among doctors using antidepressants to conduct careful and thorough suicide evaluations of their patients on treatment.

The "black box" warning may be frightening to you, however, bear in mind that untreated depression, bipolar, or other psychiatric disorders can also lead to suicide.

which include the increased use of SSRIs, alone or in combination with psychotherapy. It's very disturbing for a family to have a suicidal child. Aggressive treatment of the underlying problem causing suicidal behavior is the most valuable thing a family can do for their child to prevent this unfortunate tragedy.

Since the "black box" warning came out, many doctors have reduced or stopped prescribing antidepressants to their patients, especially primary care doctors who have less experience than psychiatrists in using these medications. However, this trend may prove to be quite dangerous for patients with mood disorders who may continue to suffer and progress in their illness without the benefit of antidepressants. Recently, the FDA considered issuing the "black box" warning on medications for seizures, which also have been found to be associated with increased suicidal behavior. A panel of experts felt that issuing the warning could have a negative effect on seizure treatment, in part based on the recent pattern of declining antidepressant use following the "black box" warnings.

All in all, the "black box" warning can be a scary concept for the public and medical community alike. Yet, for many patients, antidepressants can make the difference between a brisk recovery and terrible suffering. It is best to discuss your concerns about the warning with your doctor, and come to a reasonable treatment conclusion for your child with regard to antidepressant treatment. In many cases, it may be wiser to use the antidepressant and pay more attention to monitoring for suicidality in the child than avoid its use and risk undertreatment and other serious consequences.

For many patients, antidepressants can make the difference between a brisk recovery and terrible suffering.

56. Are there other types of antidepressant medication available to children besides the SSRIs?

Several categories of antidepressants exist in addition to the SSRIs (see Tables 15 and 17). The differences in the medications lie in their chemistry. As mentioned earlier, the three major neurotransmitters of mood disorders are serotonin, norepinephrine, and dopamine. The functions of serotonin and dopamine have already been mentioned. The neurotransmitter norepinephrine is responsible for attention, is associated with the "fight or flight" response, acts upon heart rate and blood pressure, and is involved with arousal and wakefulness. Some examples of other categories of antidepressants are ones that affect both serotonin and norepinephrine, which include venlafaxine (Effexor). There are also those that act on norepinephrine and dopamine which include bupropion (Wellbutrin). Those antidepressants that affect norepinephrine and certain types of serotonin receptors include mirtazapine (Remeron). There are antidepressants that affect the transport of serotonin in the body, which include nefazodone (Serzone) and trazodone (Desyrel). Tricyclic antidepressants (TCAs) represent one of the older categories of antidepressants. The TCAs affect primarily the neurotransmitters, serotonin and norepinephrine, and encompass a long list of medications, one of which is nortriptyline (Pamelor). Finally, monoamine oxidase inhibitors (MAOIs), also an older but highly effective antidepressant class, act by affecting the amounts of serotonin, norepinephrine, and dopamine available, and include phenylzine (Nardil).

For the patient, it may not be necessary to know how the different antidepressants work, but rather to be

Treatment

familiar with the different families of medications and be aware that your doctor may have reason to use one over the other, or choose certain combinations. Once your doctor has evaluated your child and feels a particular antidepressant is recommended, you should feel free to ask more questions about the choices.

57. If my daughter really has bipolar disorder, and is treated only for the depression, what will happen?

Many cases of bipolar disorder are unrecognized in the earlier stages of the illness. As mentioned, it often takes years for the diagnosis of BPD to be determined and the earlier presentation of the disorder in children favors depression. Furthermore, depressed children seem to experience future mania (and therefore a diagnosis of BPD) at much higher rates than adults who first experience depression. Nonetheless, it is fairly common for a depressed child with no prior diagnosis of BPD to receive treatment for depression alone. She may benefit from the treatment and make a full recovery. However, antidepressant use can cause symptoms that look like mania (manic-like symptoms) in people who have BPD as well as others who do not have BPD. Whether the antidepressant caused a "switch" to the manic symptoms of BPD (a **manic switch**) in vulnerable individuals or merely had an activating effect on an individual is a matter of debate. Usually, if your daughter is known to have BPD, antidepressant use for a depressive or mixed episode would be done only in conjunction with a mood stabilizer (see the next question for details) rather than alone. Treatment with medications for depression alone will not only be inadequate in a person with established BPD, but could

Manic switch

A situation where a patient with BPD becomes suddenly manic during a depressed episode. Antidepressants sometimes cause manic switches in vulnerable bipolar patients, especially those who are not on mood stabilizers.

make the general symptoms worse and put her at risk for a manic episode. Some researchers believe that antidepressants can encourage more rapid cycling between episodes in certain types of BPD. Furthermore, treating only the depression in a person with BPD will not eliminate the risks of future manic or mixed manic-depressive episodes. The preferred medications for BPD once mania has been documented are mood stabilizers, alone or in combination with another mood stabilizer or an antidepressant.

It's very important to give your doctor a thorough history of symptoms seen in your child as well as family history of depression or BPD to ensure that an accurate diagnosis of a depressive disorder can be made. Equally important is to keep your doctor closely updated about any changes in symptoms during the course of antidepressant treatment. Constant communication while under treatment will help your doctor determine if the antidepressant is helping your child and if other concerns are raised such as the development of manic symptoms.

58. What are mood stabilizers, and how do they work?

Mood stabilizers are the class of medications used to bring mania or hypomania of BPD back to a neutral state (see Table 18). These medicines work on the brain in various ways, but exactly how they cause mood stabilization is not entirely clear. Several theories exist on the mechanism of mood stabilizers, which include interfering with the way chemicals in the brain cells are transmitted, and/or causing changes in the activity of chemicals that can "calm down" the brain.

Traditionally, mood stabilizers have included lithium, valproic acid, and carbemazepine. The latter two of these medicines are often used to treat seizures. Doctors have recently discovered that many other medicines used to treat seizures, known as anticonvulsants, also act as mood stabilizers. A model, known as the kindling effect, has been used to explain the gradual excitement of nerve cells in the brain that eventually develops into a seizure, much the way a small burning stick evolves into a forest fire. The antiseizure medications stop seizures by increasing the activity of chemicals that calm the brain cells or decreasing the activity of chemicals that excite the brain cells. Since these medicines can also calm down the symptoms of mania, scientists feel that the kindling effect may apply to the development of mania at the level of brain cells as with seizures. Also included in this list are several other anticonvulsants seen in Table 18. The medicines used to treat hallucinations and aggression, the antipsychotic medicines, can also have mood stabilizing effects. Both the anticonvulsants and antipsychotics are used "off-label" for mood stabilization in children, although in several cases they are FDA-approved for seizure disorders and other problems. Lithium is FDA-approved for acute mania in patients over the age of 12.

Mood stabilizers may be used as single agents or in combination with other mood stabilizers to treat mania. As mentioned earlier, for depression, a mood stabilizer may be used alone or in combination with an antidepressant to achieve remission of the depressive symptoms and prevent a recurrence of either the depression or mania.

59. I've heard a lot about lithium. Isn't it "too strong" to use in children?

Lithium has been around for more than a century, and its properties for mood enhancement have been well known for a long time. It was not approved by the FDA, however, until only the last 30–40 years, due to the concerns about how to use it safely, since it could be toxic in the wrong amount. Lithium is a salt which travels into and out of nerve cells much like the naturally occurring sodium. Lithium seems to interfere with the excitement of nerve cells by its interaction with certain proteins (G-proteins), thereby "calming down" excessive cellular activity responsible for mania. When used carefully, it is an excellent mood stabilizing medicine for BPD and is still considered by many to be the gold standard for treatment of this disorder. Lithium is credited with preventing suicide in many cases of BPD. Not only is it valuable in the treatment of BPD, it is also a frequently used augmentation agent (see Question 60) for depression. People, young and old, have been helped by lithium over the years and the FDA approves it for mania in children over 12. Whether or not it is "too strong" or too risky to use in younger children in the off-label manner is a matter of debate, since untreated BPD at a young age can be a devastating illness and cause serious long-term disability, and even suicide. In such cases, tough times may call for tough measures such as lithium to control the symptoms.

Once the decision to use lithium has been made, it is still fraught with challenges. Many people (especially teenagers) dislike or can't tolerate lithium for its various side effects (see Table 20). These may include stomach upset or diarrhea, a tremor, acne, bedwetting, excessive drinking of fluids, or more serious effects such as toxicity to the thyroid gland or kidneys. Using lithium requires careful monitoring, including periodic blood tests to ensure that the level in the blood is both safe and in the therapeutic range (too much can do harm, whereas too little can do nothing but cause a few side effects), and that other parts of the body such as the thyroid and kidneys are functioning well. Careful supervision is also needed for lithium, since taking an excessive dose (especially if it is in liquid form where measurement errors are easy to make) can result in dangerous consequences. Also, caution is needed with regard to using other medicines, such as ibuprofen, which can affect the levels of lithium in the blood. People on lithium need to drink plenty of fluids to help the kidneys break down the medication properly. Young women on lithium who are sexually active need to use birth control, since the medication could cause abnormalities in a developing fetus. (This is not to say that women on lithium can't have healthy children; in pregnancy, additional measures are required for those who take lithium, to ensure a better outcome to the baby). Finally, some youngsters may not be candidates for lithium or, if they are, may require even more health supervision to avoid bad outcomes. These include children with a single kidney or kidney disorder, since lithium is broken down and excreted by the kidneys.

Some of the ways of handling side effects with lithium include starting at a low dose and increasing it slowly to allow the body time to adjust to the physical effects of the medication. Taking the medication with food and using an alternate preparation such as lithium citrate (over carbonate) or a longer acting tablet (over short acting capsule) can also be helpful to avoid stomach upset. If lithium is helping with the mood symptoms, then problems such as acne might be treated separately by the child's pediatrician or dermatologist. Suppression of the thyroid gland could be managed by replacing thyroid hormone in the form of medication known as levothyroxine. An intolerable lithium tremor is sometimes treated with low doses of blood pressure medications.

Lithium probably has one of the highest numbers of required precautions as compared to other medications in the treatment of mood disorders. Yet, when recommended, it can have a robust effect on your child's treatment and recovery. Your doctor will be the best resource for you with regard to the appropriateness of lithium in your child's treatment, and how to manage any side effects. Don't be afraid to explore the possibility of lithium, or hesitate to ask all the relevant questions.

60. What does it mean when our doctor is "augmenting" medications?

Augmentation of medication is the practice of adding a second medication, perhaps in a smaller than usual dose, to help improve the effectiveness of the first medication. An example of this would be adding a low dose of a mood stabilizer like lithium to an antidepressant to help the antidepressant do a better job in alleviating depressive symptoms. Other agents used for augmentation besides mood stabilizers include other antidepressants and thyroid hormone. Augmentation is often considered when the response of a medication is partial but not complete. Many doctors consider augmentation instead of a complete switch to another medicine.

Augmentation

The addition of a second medication to a primary one, in order to boost the effects of the first medication. Common augmentation agents for depression include lithium, thyroid hormone, and bupropion. Often a smaller dose of the augmentation agent is used to assist the primary medication.

61. What if the SSRI doesn't work? What can be done next to help the depression?

If your child continues to experience symptoms of depression after a reasonable trial of an SSRI (usually 4–8 weeks on the highest therapeutic dose), there are other options to consider. Your doctor may choose to continue that medicine and add a low dose of a mood stabilizer like lithium, or other medication, which, as previously mentioned, can augment the SSRI. Alternatively, a switch can be made to a different SSRI or class of antidepressant, such as one that acts on different neurotransmitters like norepinephrine and/or dopamine. At other times, your doctor may want to continue the SSRI and add one of the other classes of antidepressant just described.

Almost always, treatment of depression in children and adolescents requires a number of different interventions, which are not limited to medications.

Almost always, treatment of depression in children and adolescents requires a number of different interventions, which are not limited to medications. A combination of medication such as an SSRI, intensive psychotherapy of a type such as cognitive behavioral therapy, lifestyle changes such as introducing routines and exercise, school interventions, and possibly family therapy might all be part of the larger treatment plan needed to address all the aspects of a child's depression.

62. What medicines are available to treat my child's anxiety?

The discovery of SSRIs has been a major breakthrough in psychiatric treatment, especially for children. Not only are they highly effective in treating depression, but they are also beneficial in controlling

anxiety, and are much safer to use than older antidepressant medications. Often, a child psychiatrist will
use an SSRI to treat an anxious child for anxiety alone,
or for a combination of depression and anxiety. Some
other medicines that may be useful for anxiety (see
Table 13) include tricyclic antidepressants (the TCAs),
the MAOIs, diphendramine (an over-the-counter
drug), a mood stabilizer called gabapentin, and occasionally the **benzodiazepines**. An example of the latter
is valium. The benzodiazepines, while extremely helpful for panic attacks, several types of anxiety disorders,
and alcohol withdrawal, are used far less often with
children than with adults due to the long term potential for dependency and addiction and the frequent
occurrence of inappropriate, agitated, and silly behavior when used with children. Furthermore, research
studies have failed to show real benefit from benzodiazepine treatment for anxiety in the pediatric population. However, many psychiatrists in practice will
report that their child and adolescent patients are
helped tremendously by the short-term use of benzodiazepines while waiting for another treatment, like an
SSRI, to take effect. Your doctor will be able to determine what medication or combination of medicines
may be appropriate for your child.

63. Why would my doctor prescribe antipsychotic medication if my child does not have schizophrenia?

Traditionally, antipsychotic medications (or simply,
antipsychotics) have been used to treat psychosis. Psychosis describes a constellation of experiences that
includes auditory and visual hallucinations, false beliefs
known as delusions, disorganized thinking or behavior,

Benzodiazepines
A class of medica-
tions used to treat
anxiety, seizures,
insomnia, or alcohol
withdrawal. These
medicines act upon a
set of neurotransmit-
ters that cause calm-
ing and sedation.

Psychosis describes a constellation of experiences that includes auditory and visual hallucinations, false beliefs known as delusions, disorganized thinking or behavior, other problems with reality testing traditionally associated with the illness schizophrenia.

and other problems with reality testing traditionally associated with the illness schizophrenia. Schizophrenia is a chronic, disabling disorder that presents with a variety of problems, some of which include psychosis and impairments in social or occupational functioning. Since their discovery, antipsychotics substantially improved the lives of people with schizophrenia. More recently, antipsychotics have been used to treat other illnesses besides schizophrenia. Certain cases of depression or mania present with psychosis and these are helped tremendously by antipsychotics. In some mood disordered patients who have social withdrawal or poor communication, these medications can help improve such symptoms. Antipsychotics are extremely helpful in reducing aggressive behaviors in children and are commonly used in lower doses (than used for psychosis) to help with aggression. Psychiatrists and pediatricians often consider antipsychotics to treat aggression seen in youngsters with developmental disorders such as **autism**. Antipsychotics also have mood stabilizing properties, as discussed in an earlier question, and may help reduce symptoms of mania much like one of the more classic mood stabilizers. Finally, in children who have Tourette's disorder, an illness characterized by tics (harmless, but annoying repetitive movements and/or inappropriate, involuntary verbal comments), antipsychotic medication has been found to substantially reduce these symptoms.

Doctors are cautious about using antipsychotics, primarily because they pose a risk for some rare, but concerning complications. These include a life-threatening disorder characterized by muscle rigidity, high fever, and some other worrisome symptoms (neuroleptic malignant syndrome, or NMS) and the possibility of developing an irreversible condition over time that is

Autism

Also known as autistic disorder in the *DSM*. Autism is a neurodevelopmental disorder that begins in infancy and early childhood that is characterized by profound deficits in social functioning and communication, restricted interests, and/or repetitive behaviors.

characterized by abnormal movements (tardive dyskinesia). Again, it is rare to develop either of these problems on antipsychotics but, because of the seriousness of these conditions, psychiatrists will closely monitor any child on an antipsychotic medicine for the development of these side effects. Other strategies to minimize future risks and side effects from the drugs include using the lowest necessary dose and raising the dose slowly. Also, discontinuing an antipsychotic medicine after a period of time if symptoms of illness have subsided has also been helpful to reduce the long term risks for developing tardive dyskinesia. Recently, it has also been shown that the atypical antipsychotic medicines can cause significant weight gain, possibly increase the risk of developing diabetes, and possibly accelerate the development of cardiovascular disease, all of which may lead to future health issues. As a result, doctors are more cautious than ever about when to prescribe antipsychotics, how long to prescribe them, and which choices are made among different antipsychotics (some agents carry a lower risk than others with regard to weight gain and diabetes). Doctors may perform periodic tests, which include monitoring height and weight and checking your child's blood for high sugar, as well as other blood tests. Usually the doctor will also perform an examination, known as the **AIMS (Abnormal Involuntary Movement Scale) test**, every few months to assess for any developing abnormal movements. More frequent, but less harmful side effects of antipsychotic medications include sedation, dry mouth, constipation, increased appetite, a feeling of inner restlessness and outer fidgetiness known as **akathisia**, acute muscle spasms and other problems where the muscles seem to "freeze up" or slow down (**dystonia**).

Treatment

AIMS test

Also known as the Abnormal Involuntary Movement Scale. This is an examination done by a doctor or other trained health professional to test for tardive dyskinesia. It is a brief exam that is recorded onto a rating scale, and performed about every few months to monitor for the development of tardive dyskinesia.

Akathisia

A feeling of inner restlessness often caused by medications such as antipsychotics or antidepressants. Outer signs of akathisia include motor restlessness such as fidgetiness.

Dystonia

Also known as a dystonic reaction. The sudden or gradual development of uncomfortable and possibly painful spasms of muscle groups in the neck, eyes, extremities, or muscles involved in speech and breathing. The problem develops within a few hours or days after a medication, especially an antipsychotic is started or increased in dose. Dystonia often responds to anticholinergic medications, or to removal of the offending agent.

Two classes of antipsychotic medications are available. The older class, known as the traditional or typical antipsychotic agents, primarily affects the neurotransmitter, dopamine, and has more side effects on the nervous system. The newer class of antipsychotic agents, known as the atypical antipsychotics or second generation antipsychotics, affects dopamine as well as serotonin and has fewer side effects on the nervous system. The atypical antipsychotics are now used far more often than the traditional antipsychotics, especially in children. Even though they have a better side effect profile, occasionally doctors will still have to address some undesirable, but usually harmless, side effects, such as akathesia and the "freezing" effect on muscles. Both of these problems can usually be managed by switching to a different medicine, or by adding low doses of another type of medicine, known as **anticholinergic medications** to the treatment regimen. Atypical antipsychotics can be quite valuable in treating children with a mood disorder but, like certain other medications, require a high level of supervision with use. You are encouraged to further discuss with your doctor how this type of medicine might benefit your child.

Anticholinergic medications

A family of medications acting upon the neurotransmitter, acetylcholine, which helps reverse some of the side effects such as acute muscle spasms and restlessness caused by psychotropic medications. A commonly used anticholinergic medications is benztropine (trade name Cogentin).

64. How should medications be administered to children?

In general, parents should carefully supervise their children when it comes to medications. The maturity of your child will guide your approach, of course. Younger children, such as those under 12, should not dispense from the pill bottle(s) themselves, but rather an adult should remove the pill or capsule and give it to them. Direct observation of the child, where you watch your child taking the medicine with water, is always a good idea. If there is any concern that your child is not swallowing the pill or is spitting it out, you should ask to check her mouth after she takes it. Some medications, like fluoxetine or lithium, might be given in liquid form if swallowing pills is an issue. It is especially important that **you** measure and dispense your child's liquid medicine to them, as any mistakes in measurement could lead to overdosage.

It's a little trickier with teenagers and medications. Adolescents are always trying to do things for themselves and value their independence. They might feel insulted that their parents are giving them their pills when it is something they could do on their own. Parents may want to appease their teen by letting him take his own pills, or they may feel he is mature enough to handle it alone and it would be one less thing for the adults to remember. Here is where the trouble often begins. Many teens (and adults) are forgetful and miss doses of medications. This is especially true in the morning, when everyone is rushing to get out the door to school on time and often neglecting to make time for breakfast or other important things. Furthermore, almost all teenagers have some ambivalence about taking medications, since taking the pills means that they have surrendered control of their own bodies. When left on their own to take medicine with such ambivalence, it is not uncommon for teenagers to stop the medication unbeknownst to the parents. In order to prevent such a situation from happening in the first place, it is best to start out supervising your teen when taking medicine. This is not to deny that some teenagers are highly responsible and trustworthy with regard to self-medicating. However, you should ask your child how she feels about taking the medicine and keep her involved in the process of administering the medicine. You should also discuss with your doctor how best to approach ongoing supervision.

65. Are there any monitoring tests my son will have to undergo once he is being treated with psychiatric medications?

Your son may need certain evaluations once he is on medications. These may include blood tests to see that the body is functioning well and that certain abilities of the body are not being impaired by the medications. The mood stabilizers may require measuring blood levels of the drug to make sure that amount of medication in the body is within the range that is safe and also therapeutic. Other laboratory tests to monitor depend of the type of medication that is being used. Lithium use requires monitoring the tests for kidney function and thyroid function. Other mood stabilizers like valproic acid and many atypical antipsychotic medications will require monitoring the ability of the body to make healthy blood cells and other components of the blood. Tests monitoring how the liver functions may be checked periodically, as most psychotropic medications are broken down by the liver (the others are handled by the kidneys). A pregnancy test and/or a urine drug test may also be done to make sure it is safe to give your child medications and ascertain whether other problems like substance abuse are complicating the presentation of illness. An electrocardiogram (EKG) may be needed to monitor the heart's ability to function normally while on certain medications.

The mood stabilizers may require measuring blood levels of the drug to make sure that amount of medication in the body is within the range that is safe and also therapeutic.

Other tests that are often monitored include periodic height, weight, heart rate, and blood pressure, as these may be affected by various medications. Some of these tests may be performed by the psychiatrist, and others may be requested through your child's pediatrician.

Your doctor will let you know more specifically which tests and examinations need to be followed while your child is on medication.

66. How long does it take to see a response to treatment, once medication is started for depression or mania?

The time needed for a treatment response depends on the disorder itself, the circumstances around the illness, and the medicine used. Unlike the immediate results seen when treating ADHD with psychostimulant medications, it usually takes longer to see improvements on medication with a mood disorder. The time ranges from days to weeks, and possibly even several months. This delay is due to several reasons. First, some medications, such as the SSRIs, cause biochemical changes in the way the brain and liver make and use proteins and other substances involved with mood. These chemical changes can take a few weeks to occur. Second, other factors, such as stressful life situations or environmental factors that are contributing to the mood disorder are usually not resolved immediately and can interfere with a medication's ability to treat symptoms effectively. Third, without realizing it, children with mood disorders and their families often engage in self-defeating habits or patterns of behavior that cause or perpetuate symptoms of the disorder, regardless of whether medication is being used. Even

115

after medicine is started, other treatments such as individual and family therapy are usually needed to address these dysfunctional tendencies. As we all know, undoing negative habits can take time. Finally, certain disorders are episodic and will take a natural course of improving over time despite treatment. Examples of this include resolution of a hypomanic episode on its own within a few days, or a depressive episode within 6–10 months. Thus, even if the medication never has an impact on the disorder (i.e., there is no treatment response), the symptoms may resolve within a certain time frame. All these factors really illustrate the complexity in evaluating treatment response, and how medications alone are not the only consideration in determining if and how long it takes for a child's symptoms to improve.

It can seem rather delayed to have to wait so long when every day, even every minute of suffering, can be highly intolerable both to the child and her family. Sometimes, the doctor can temporarily add another medicine to "jump start" the treatment, such as giving a hypnotic medication for sleep or a benzodiazepine for severe anxiety and agitation. Then, as the primary treatment such as an antidepressant or mood stabilizer has had more time to take effect, the additional agents can be tapered off or discontinued. Being in a supportive treatment with a competent therapist (whether it is your psychiatrist or another mental health professional working with your psychiatrist) is also helpful for a child and family to weather the delay of a medication taking effect.

67. Once a child starts taking medications for a mood disorder, can she become "addicted"?

Addiction is a frequently used term to describe behavior that seeks to use drugs for reasons of physical or emotional need. An addict must use that drug because he is in the habit of doing so, or to prevent/treat a physical or psychological reaction (**withdrawal**) that has occurred when the drug is not in that person's body. The term "addict" is often perceived as judgmental and generally invokes images of street drugs. Many parents are concerned about using psychotropic medications in children because they attribute information they have on illegal drugs and addiction to all drugs, including those that are prescribed. Some parents equate all medicines with street drugs. In doing so, they may also fear that prescribed medications can cause the same type of negative consequences as illicit substances.

In reality, few medicines used to treat children are addictive. The terms more appropriate to use in talking about medications are **tolerance** (a situation where higher and higher amounts of the medication are needed in order to produce the same effect), and **dependence** (a situation where a pattern of behavior seeking out the medicine has been established, and possibly that the body has a developed a physical requirement for the medication without which negative physical symptoms would occur). The psychostimulants, medications used to treat attention deficit hyperactivity disorder, are a group of medicines to which a child could become tolerant, and the benzodiazepines, used infrequently with younger children but occasionally with teenagers for anxiety, sleep, or

Addiction

According to the National Institute on Drug Abuse (NIDA), drug addiction is a brain disease characterized by compulsive drug seeking and use despite harmful consequences.

Withdrawal

A physical or psychological reaction that occurs when a drug of abuse is discontinued. Craving or drug seeking is generally associated with withdrawal.

The term "addict" is often perceived as judgmental and generally invokes images of street drugs.

Tolerance

The need for higher doses of a medication to have the same effect after prolonged use.

Dependence

Continued need to use a drug without which a physical or psychological reaction would occur. Often a pattern of seeking the drug has been established.

Treatment

severe mania, could cause dependence. Careful and responsible use of these prescribed medications generally does not cause addiction. However, it has been shown that stimulants, benzodiazepines, and other prescription medicines, which include sleeping pills, narcotic pain relievers, over-the-counter diet pills containing amphetamine, and cough medicines containing codeine, can be abused and their use lead to future dependency. For this reason, a number of these medications are considered "controlled" substances in many states and regulated carefully by the Drug Enforcement Agency and pharmacies.

The scientific literature fails to demonstrate addiction to mood stabilizers, antipsychotics, or antidepressants. However, the public perception of these medicines often suggests otherwise, as noted in a major survey done in London in the 1990s by Professor Robert Priest, where more than three-quarters of 2,000 adults surveyed thought that antidepressants were addictive. It has also been been noted that, even though antidepressants, mood stabilizers, and antipsychotics are not addictive, stopping some of these medicines abruptly after a long period of treatment has been known to cause temporary unpleasant reactions. These reactions, previously called a withdrawal syndrome, are now referred to as a **discontinuation syndrome.** The discontinuation syndrome includes uncomfortable neurologic, gastroenterologic, and/or flu-like symptoms. Experts acknowledge a distinction between drug and alcohol withdrawal and the discontinuation syndrome in that the latter generally has a less severe symptom profile and a lack of drug craving or drug seeking behavior upon removal of the medication.

Discontinuation syndrome

An unpleasant bodily experience occurring within a few days to weeks of abruptly stopping a medication or missing doses, especially the SSRIs or other antidepressants. The experience often includes flu-like symptoms such as headache, dizziness, nausea, and other neurologic or gastrointestinal complaints, as well as possible mood and anxiety symptoms.

You are encouraged to speak further with your doctor about concerns you may have about addiction and pre-scribed medications. Sometimes having a family member or friend with a drug addiction and related bad experiences can influence parents' attitudes toward medications. Clarifying the issue for yourself is very important and may help alleviate anxieties about addiction raised by including psychotropic medications in your child's treatment.

68. What if my child uses drugs or alcohol while taking psychotropic medication?

It is actually very common for teenagers (or preteens) who are suffering from emotional problems to drink, smoke, or take illegal drugs. For example, alcohol can help calm feelings of agitation or unease, as can ciga-rettes or marijuana. Cocaine or amphetamines can make someone who is depressed feel happy or ener-gized, and heroin can make someone feeling too active become calm. Many other drugs have properties that can counteract undesirable feelings or behaviors. At times, **substance abuse** (ongoing, overuse, or misuse of a drug) can be an effort to "numb" intense feelings, or make a chronically bad feeling more tolerable. Accord-ing to the National Institute for Drug Abuse (NIDA), children and adolescents are most vulnerable to drug abuse during periods of transition in their lives, such as moving between elementary and middle school, or between middle and high school. In addition, NIDA identifies multiple risk and protective factors, the imbalance of which can lead to drug abuse and addic-tion. Some of the risk factors for teens include peer pressure, biological vulnerability (i.e., a strong family

Substance abuse

Repeated use of illicit drugs that leads to negative consequences.

history and/or genetic predisposition) to drug abuse, easy access to drugs, a chaotic home life, poorly controlled psychiatric symptoms, or a combination of these factors. Undertreated mood symptoms, along with the persistence of some of the risk factors mentioned, could motivate your child to use drugs or alcohol despite being on treatment with psychotropic medications. Unfortunately, it's almost always dangerous to mix drugs or alcohol with medications. Like psychotropic medications, alcohol and illicit drugs such as marijuana, cocaine, amphetamines, etc., also affect the brain. Many drugs, including alcohol, when mixed with antidepressants or mood stabilizers, will have an additive effect and further impact the brain and nervous system, leading to dullness or agitation, poor judgment, excessive sleepiness, unusual behavioral reactions, or even a loss of consciousness. Combining medication and alcohol or drugs, even if only occasionally or in small amounts, can be not only dangerous, but life threatening.

If your son or daughter is drinking or using illegal drugs while taking prescribed medications, he or she needs help.

If your son or daughter is drinking or using illegal drugs while taking prescribed medications, he or she needs help. The first step would be to address the issue in treatment with your doctor, and consider what other strategies need to be considered in the larger psychiatric treatment plan. Some clinicians are able to include drug testing, prescription of medications specific to the treatment of drug addiction, and/or integrate psychotherapies specific to the treatment of drug addiction. If your doctor does not feel equipped to manage drug abuse in the psychiatric treatment, then a referral might be given for another professional or program that specializes in the treatment of substance abuse. The government-run agency, SAMHSA, offers Internet listings by state for substance abuse programs available to the public (see Question 100). Many inpatient psychiatric programs also handle cases of **dual diagnosis**, where both substance abuse and other psychiatric problems have been identified. Community-based organizations such as Alcoholics Anonymous (AA) and Narcotics Anonymous (NA) may serve as resources for information as well as support groups for drug and alcohol problems affecting teenagers and their families (see Question 100). Finally, the NIDA also has some free publications online for teenagers as well as caregivers that provide information about drug abuse (see Question 100).

Dual diagnosis

The situation of having both a psychiatric disorder such as a mood disorder or schizophrenia and a substance abuse disorder.

Treatment

69. Is taking medication for depression or bipolar disorder a lifelong commitment?

It is daunting for most parents to think that their child will need to take medication for the rest of her life. Many chronic conditions require a long term commitment to medications, and some do not. A mood disorder may fall into either of these categories. What will influence the need for long term medication is whether a pattern of recurrence exists. For depression, a first episode may not tell you if it will recur, although many cases of depression are recurrent. In general, if a medication helps to reduce or eliminate symptoms of a depressed, manic, or mixed episode, it should be continued for at least a certain period of time. In cases of depression, experts suggest a minimum of 6–12 months of treatment with the antidepressant medication before discontinuing it. If the depression recurs soon after stopping the medication, then a longer course of treatment is indicated, and possibly a continuous treatment course. Bipolar disorder has a somewhat different set of recommendations than depression. More continuous treatment with a mood stabilizer is generally advised, with possible intermittent use of other medicines such as antidepressants, depending on the frequency of depressive or manic episodes. Experts suggest a minimum of 12–24 months of treatment with a mood stabilizer for the treatment of a manic episode. As with antidepressants, after the mood stabilizer is discontinued, if symptoms of the illness return, the medicine will need to be restarted and a plan for longer treatment may be needed.

Time will often help determine how long your child should be taking medications for his mood disorder. Like other chronic illnesses of childhood such as asthma or seizures, a mood disorder may require extended treatment. The decision to continue medications over time is of the utmost importance for your child's long term health and well-being. Ongoing discussions with your doctor about it are recommended, and may provide the reassurance needed by parents around the stress and uncertainty of their child's future while living with depression or BPD.

70. Will taking medications change my child's personality?

In the 1980s, a popular book written by psychiatrist Peter Kramer, entitled *Listening to Prozac* described the dramatic impact that fluoxetine had upon the lives of the depressed people taking it. The SSRIs were relatively new at that time and the improvements observed on them were so profound, it was as if those people had a change of personality. Adults whose entire lives took on the negative characteristics of their depression were transformed and had a completely different, more positive outlook on everything once on treatment. While this kind of transformation can occur (I myself once treated a teenager with disabling BPD who went from being a terror to a delight once he was placed on the appropriate treatments), it is not often in a way that the essence of the child is altered. Rather, medications will usually modify aspects of your child to ones that are better functioning or more adaptive than before the treatment. These aspects can include attitudes as well as behaviors. Occasionally, a family may feel that a child has lost her "spark" with treatment. If medication is causing your child to be "someone else" and the result makes other people in the family uncomfortable, then you may want to discuss that further with your doctor to determine if the treatment is the best choice available.

71. My daughter, who has bipolar illness, wants to be an artist and does her best artwork when she is having a manic episode. Will mood stabilizing medicines dull her creativity?

This question is a continuation of the previous one where a parent is concerned that the "essence" of the child" is changed by medications. A common complaint that many artists suffering from BPD have is the reduction in creativity experienced when placed on medications, especially lithium. Yet, many famous creative people, felt to have mood disorders, have had periods of low productivity and even terrible endings to their lives by suicide from the lack of or undertreatment of their illnesses. Popular culture tends to romanticize certain emotional disorders and frequently attributes the creativity of artists suffering from these illnesses as a product of their mood disordered states. It is as if those people, if cured of their symptoms, would be less of who they really are. A number of well-regarded psychiatric professionals have written about the topic of creativity and mood disorders. They found that a relationship between the two may certainly exist, but often artists such as painters and writers who were evaluated for the problem, did their best work or were highly productive when their disordered symptoms were resolved or under control, rather than during the acute episodes of the illness. It has also been noted in the literature that artists with BPD who are treated with medications frequently have difficulty with taking their medicines consistently and use the potential loss of creativity to justify their discontinuation. At times, their concerns are legitimate as a number of mood stabilizing medications can affect the way the brain processes and communicates information and may interfere with their work. Yet, at other times, the medicines may not interfere with their ability to produce high quality work at all. In such cases, stopping the medicines may be an expression of their ambivalence about the role of medication in their treatment.

Your daughter's talents should be recognized as a part of who she is and not merely a derivative of an emotional state she may be experiencing some of the time. Also, you and she may want to explore, with other creative individuals and in psychotherapy, different ways to access her creativity that would help her pursue her dreams of being an artist. Since mood stabilizing medication is a fundamental part of the treatment for BPD, if one medicine appears to interfere with her thinking or her creative work, then an alternative choice should be considered. Over the course of her lifetime, the chances of success with her talents are far improved with good, consistent treatment of her BPD.

72. Will medicines used to treat my son's depression affect his ability to think clearly in school?

This question, like the last one, asks about performance ability while on medication but also addresses a different issue, i.e., discriminating between a symptom of the mood disorder and a side effect of the medication. Many children who are depressed may have problems thinking clearly or concentrating as a symptom of the depression or other psychiatric disorder. It's also possible that the medicine used to treat the psychiatric symptoms is causing cognitive dulling (thinking more slowly or in a cloudy way) or poor concentration as a side effect of the psychiatric medication. However, not all children have the same experience: whereas one medicine may be sedating or dulling for one child, it may be activating (making more alert and active) and improving the concentration for another. Several of the antidepressants can make people feel tired during the day, which could contribute to cloudy thinking or sleepiness during the school day. Several of the mood stabilizers, and some other classes of medicines, such as the atypical antipsychotics, can also be very dulling or clouding. This is especially true in the first few weeks of starting the medicine. Often, this side effect can be reduced by either giving the medicine in the evening or at night, giving the higher doses toward the evening (if it's a medicine given more than once a day), or possibly raising the dose more slowly so the body has a chance to get used to the effects. If those strategies don't work, your doctor may choose to change the medicine altogether and find one that has a more favorable side effect profile.

As mentioned, some medicines are more activating and may be a better choice for a child whose depressive symptoms render him "dull" or tired. An antidepressant, such as fluoxetine, may be preferred over another, such as sertraline, for the side effect of sedation. If your son has symptoms of ADHD in addition to the mood symptoms, it might be helpful for him to be taking a psychostimulant medication which is known to help concentration and thinking, and often "wakes" people up. Other alternatives may exist to address the problem of cognitive dulling and/or sedation. A thorough discussion with your doctor about the symptoms of your son's illness and treatment options is recommended to find the best choices for him.

73. Will my child be "labeled" negatively by others once he starts taking medications?

It's hard to predict the reaction of a community to a child who needs medications. If your child is in a special school or program with other children who also take medications and teachers with experience in working with such children, it may not be an issue. However, more often than not, a child can feel different from her peers because of psychiatric illness and/or the need for medication. Both adults and children have reactions to the idea of medications. Adults, such as parents of your child's classmates, friends, relatives, or teachers may have biases about medications. Some may believe that medicines are not appropriate for children, or are overused without understanding the basis for their use. Others may feel medicines serve as a "crutch" or substitute for good parenting, and can be judgmental about the need for medication. On occasion, adults can believe that prescribed medications are like illegal drugs, which can be addictive and dangerous (see also Question 67). Children can be cruel and mocking of others who behave differently than they do, or make those who need medication feel ashamed. All these assumptions and reactions by others suggest either fear or a lack of knowledge about the medicines and/or psychiatric disorders.

You may find ways to handle the problem of depression or bipolar disorder in the public setting in a manner that is sensitive to your child. This may include giving him his medications at home to avoid his feeling "scrutinized" at school, which may happen if the child needs to see the school nurse to receive a dose of medicine during the day. However, the larger issue is really overcoming the shame often associated with an emotional disorder, and the embarrassment of the treatment. Feeling well-informed and being able to educate the community on the disorder and its treatments are effective ways of addressing the stigma of the illness or the medicines, and empowering you and your family. Participating in your school's parent-teacher association and initiating discussion on the topics of psychiatric illness and treatments, are important ways of bringing the community "up to speed" on the issues that your child and others are experiencing. Also, speaking with teachers or making a presentation about mental health and illness to a class in school may help reduce stigma in your community. Your local chapters of the National Association for the Mentally

Ill (NAMI), Mental Health America (MHA), the American Psychiatric Association (APA) or American Academy of Child and Adolescent Psychiatry (AACAP) may be able to help identify mental health professionals and patient advocates in the community who are willing to help in the process of educating teachers and students on psychiatric disorders and treatments as well.

74. Our doctor recently started my son on medication and we can't stand the side effects. We want to stop it. Is there a way we should do that?

Before you discontinue any medication, you should always inform your doctor that you're thinking of stopping it and find out if other options exist.

Before you discontinue any medication, you should always inform your doctor that you're thinking of stopping it and find out if other options exist. In prior questions and answers, I've reviewed some strategies that could be tried to minimize unpleasant side effects. These include slowing down the schedule to increase the dose (titration) of a new medicine, changing the delivery method of the medicine to a more tolerable one, changing to a different medication or, if the medicine alleviates the symptoms for which it is prescribed, adding on another medication to counteract the side effect of the first might be considered.

Sometimes the doctor and family will mutually agree to stop the medicine, in which case it's important to do so carefully. Don't stop any medication suddenly unless directed by your doctor. Doing so can sometimes cause some very unpleasant reactions, known as a discontinuation syndrome (see also Question 67). For example, stopping an antidepressant abruptly rather than tapering it off over a few days can make the patient feel physically ill as if she has the flu, or it can even trigger agitation or hypomanic symptoms. Suddenly stopping an antipsychotic medicine from a therapeutic dose may trigger a period of abnormal movements, again avoided with a gradual tapering schedule.

A common situation occurs where a parent reduces the dose of the child's medication without telling the doctor in the hopes of minimizing a side effect. This is especially true with sedating medicines. However, you should realize that a reduced dose may not help treat the problem for which the medication was given in the first place and it could be a waste of time to take it at all in a **subtherapeutic dose**. Again, it's best to speak with your doctor about the fact that you're thinking of reducing or discontinuing your child's medication and come up with a plan that you're all comfortable with and likely to continue.

75. My teenaged son refuses to take medication for his bipolar disorder... what can I do?

You are describing a frustrating, yet not uncommon scenario for families with teenagers struggling with BPD. It will be fairly important to understand the nature of your son's refusal. (See also Questions 93 and 94 that deal with hiding the medicines and skipping appointments.) Sometimes, it's a matter of knowing if the side effects of the medication are the reason to reject it. Your doctor may be able to suggest some alternative medicines, or different ways of taking the ones prescribed, to address intolerable side effects. If the medicine is beneficial but the side effects can't be

Subtherapeutic dose

An amount of medication below what is needed to be effective in treating the symptoms for which it is prescribed. The amount of medication that is effective is called the therapeutic dose or therapeutic window (if a range of doses is therapeutic).

reduced through modifications or changes in how they are administered, there may be other ways to address them, such as adding other treatments or behavioral changes for things such as acne, weight gain, or bed-wetting.

I've known parents who wanted to "slip" their child's medication into food or drinks so that the child wouldn't realize it. Not only is this a bad idea, but it might do more harm than good. The exact dose could be altered and an amount other than prescribed could be given if your child eats more or less food than expected. Some medicines are not meant to be crushed or broken but swallowed whole; crushing or breaking certain capsules or specialized tablets could result in the medication being delivered into the body in an incorrect way and having little effect on the child. Fur-thermore, putting medicine into the food surrepti-tiously violates the trust between you and your child. In hospitals, giving medicines to patients, even chil-dren, without their knowledge, is considered highly unethical. It gives all of you the message that you can't trust the child and the child can't trust you, a poor foundation for any relationship.

If medication refusal is based on a struggle for "con-trol," it's more challenging. This is often the reason for many youngsters, especially teenagers, to refuse medi-cines. Engaging your son in a dialogue about the dis-order and its treatment is a necessary part of treatment. Educating yourselves as a family on BPD and the treatment options is an essential step in the process of making the appropriate choices toward recovery. In some ways, having BPD and refusing medication is not that different from a teenager who has diabetes and refuses prescribed insulin. The family will need to do everything it can to help the youngster understand the nature of the illness and work toward accepting the appropriate treatment. You and your doctor will need to consider different approaches to this problem. Sometimes you may need to be patient and keep encouraging your son to consider the medication for a period of time while other aspects of treatment are being pursued, such as **psychoeducation** and psychotherapy. At other times, you might not want to allow the time, given the suffering and possible risks that are taking place with the illness untreated. Sometimes parents may need to provide disincentives to continued medication refusal such as loss of privileges or other consequences. The ultimate disincentive to medication refusal in the context of very poor functioning is, of course, hospitalization. While this strategy is coercive and generally not preferred, avoiding the hospital can provide a source of motivation in the treatment for some individuals.

Speaking with other parents of children with BPD is often helpful and appreciated as a source of support for families with a child who refuses treatment. Family-driven organizations can serve as important resources in the struggle to live with BPD, and those who have similar experiences with their children might be able to shed some perspective on ways to improve the situation.

76. Our daughter is feeling a lot better, and her symptoms of depression have resolved. When can we stop the medications?

Even without treatment, studies show that a depressive episode often has a natural course and will resolve, on

Treatment

Psychoeducation
Patient education through written materials, other media, or discussion on topics relevant to psychiatric illness and treatment.

average, within 8 months. However, allowing "nature to take its course" is not always in the best interest of your daughter, as the depression will frequently cost her considerably in school, family and social relationships, and possibly her own safety. Furthermore, an episode can last far longer than what is considered "average" and create a much greater toll on both the child and family. Medications will often shorten and improve the symptoms of the depressive episode more quickly than would occur without treatment and help your daughter function better at home and in school. Patients will often want to stop taking their medications once they feel better. This is true not only with psychiatric problems, but most medical problems, including infections, diabetes, high blood pressure, and many others. Even if the illness is one that can resolve with a short course of treatment, such as an infection requiring antibiotics, it is still important to complete the full 10 days or more of medication despite feeling well after two or three days of therapy. The reason for this is that the illness could recur if the treatment is incomplete. Similarly, a depressive episode can resolve within a few weeks or months on appropriate antidepressant treatment, but the risk of a **relapse** (of symptoms in a short period of time) or **recurrence** (return of symptoms after a longer period of time, generally after an episode has resolved) are high if the medications are stopped too soon. If your daughter has experienced multiple depressive episodes, the treatment recommendation could be longer than the minimum 6–12 months on antidepressant medication advised by experts for a first-time episode of depression.

If your daughter has been diagnosed with BPD, experts suggest treating an episode of mania for 12–24 months to prevent the symptoms from returning. This

Patients will often want to stop taking their medications once they feel better.

Relapse

A situation where the symptoms of depression return within a short time of improvement, usually, between 2 weeks and 2 months of the improvement.

Recurrence

A situation where a new episode of depression occurs after a first episode resolves, usually after 2 months or more of improvement.

recommendation would be further modified if a history of repeated episodes of mood disturbance (either mania, depression, or a mixed state) exists. Using the analogy of other medical illnesses such as diabetes or high blood pressure, the treatment of BPD, which frequently has a chronic pattern of mania and/or depression, more continuous use of medication is usually needed to prevent recurrences.

It's not easy to take medications for long period of time. However, the benefits of doing so may be worthwhile. This discussion is encouraged with your treating doctor, who will be able to help you determine the exact duration of your daughter's treatment with medications.

77. How are sleep problems associated with mood disorders treated in children?

Sleep problems in children are common among both healthy and emotionally troubled youngsters. First, we should review sleep problems of emotionally healthy children and adolescents. Very young children can have easily disrupted sleep at night as part of their brain immaturity. Usually by school age, a stable sleep pattern is established. Even for children in good health, problems falling or staying asleep can occur. Often, the difficulty is related to an inconsistent bedtime or rising time in the mornings. A frequent problem among teenagers is the habit of staying up late at night, then needing to sleep late the next day. This results in a shift in the **sleep-wake cycle**, which is not really a problem with sleep, but rather a problem with the times at which sleep is occurring. When a teenager

Sleep-wake cycle
The biological pattern that occurs every 24 hours of sleep followed by wakefulness.

needs to report to school on time and participate in class during the week, the shift in the sleep-wake cycle doesn't work out so well for him. The solution to this problem is for the teen to go to bed at the same time every night, and get up at the same time in the morning. This is surprisingly simple but often challenging to accomplish, given the competing interests of homework, a social life, television, video games, or the Internet. Another reason for sleep trouble can be the consumption of stimulating substances such as chocolate or caffeine (e.g., soda, tea, or coffee) or a substance that disturbs sleep such as alcohol or cigarettes in evening, or at bedtime. Eliminating these items from the diet later in the day may help with **insomnia**. Drinking too much liquid after dinner can disturb sleep by requiring more frequent bathroom trips at night, or even bedwetting accidents. Restricting fluid intake after a certain hour in the evening, may help with such a problem. Certain activities that are invigorating or over-stimulating, such as heavy exercise, watching violent movies or TV shows, or playing violent video games, can cause a child to "wake up" at night and are best avoided close to bedtime. Helping your child or teenager maintain a **sleep diary** for 1–2 weeks can help better characterize the problems with sleep. You can then review the sleep diary with your doctor to address areas that can be improved.

Children with mood disorders have the same challenges but, in addition, can experience trouble with sleep related to the symptoms of depression, mania, or both. Depression is frequently associated with difficulty falling or staying asleep (insomnia) or excessive need for sleep (**hypersomnia**). Mania is often characterized by little need for sleep. Treatment in the form of psychotherapy, psychoeducation, and/or

Insomnia

Difficulty in falling asleep or staying asleep.

Sleep diary

A written record describing several days' worth of sleep and wake times at night, daytime naps, and total number of hours of sleep every day.

Hypersomnia

Sleeping in excess of what is normally expected for one's age.

medication of the depression and mania itself, can lead to improvement in sleep difficulties, although usually the improvements in sleep are seen well after the mood improves. Some medicines used to help depression and mania, such as antidepressants and mood stabilizers, can be sedating so, if chosen wisely, and given in the evening or at night, may help induce sleep at a reasonable hour. Occasionally, your child's doctor may choose to use a class of medicines known as hypnotics (otherwise known as sleeping pills) which include benzodiazepines, (a class of anti-anxiety medication), zolpidem and other newer sleeping pills, trazadone (an antidepressant often used in low doses), or diphenhydramine, (a sedating, over-the-counter medicine used for allergies and other purposes) to help with sleep. Unlike with adults, sleeping pills are used with more caution in children and adolescents, and often only short term (i.e., a few days or weeks) to temporarily help your child get back on track with sleep until the general mood symptoms improve. The use of such medicines is usually in combination with the medicines used to treat the mood disorder. Some doctors avoid prescribing sleep medications in children as a number of these medicines may be habit forming or may cause further agitation or undesirable behaviors in children. The choices of medications to address poor sleep, along with maintaining healthy sleep habits, are all important in the discussion to have with your doctor in treating your child's mood disorder.

78. Can diet and exercise cure my child's depression?

Finding a "cure" for depression suggests a quick-fix, which at this time is a tall order not easily achieved by any one treatment. However, studies have shown that a moderate to vigorous amount of exercise can improve mood, at least temporarily. Exercise is likely to have a positive impact on a depressed child or teenager and aid in the general recovery from symptoms although it alone, without other treatment, will likely be ineffective to resolve the depressive episode. For the majority of youngsters who have only transient symptoms of low mood, in contrast to those with clinical depression, the effects of exercise is probably more dramatic. Other benefits of exercise for those suffering from mood disorders include weight management, relieving boredom, and encouraging social situations.

In the matter of diet, it is harder to make conclusions with regard to depression. Dieting and overeating have been associated with depression, although it's difficult to interpret this information since those who diet or overeat may have concerns about their weight which are related to poor self esteem and low mood.

On the other hand, helping your child establish a balanced, nutritious diet will set the stage for good physical health which will aid mental health. Involve your pediatrician in your child's treatment for mood disorder and explore how you can achieve a healthy diet and exercise plan for you child.

79. I don't believe in traditional medicines. Are there alternative treatments that I can give my depressed child?

Alternative therapies encompass a variety of treatments. A few examples include the use of herbs, nutritional supplements, massage, aromatherapy, acupuncture, yoga, hypnosis, or other healing practices outside of Western medicine. If you don't accept a treatment advised by a medical doctor, but instead use one of the "non-traditional" ones in place of that treatment, it is considered an **alternative treatment**. An example of alternative treatment would be to take an herb such as St. John's Wort instead of an antidepressant medication. However, some of the "non-traditional" treatments are frequently used in conjunction with more "traditional" treatments, in which case they are classified as **complementary treatment**. An example of complementary treatment would be to use hypnosis along with anti-anxiety medication to overcome panic attacks. A popular nutritional supplement, the omega-3 fatty acids (fish oils), is gaining popularity as a complementary treatment (also called an "add-on" treatment in some circles) with psychotropic medications or other treatments. A small but significant study done by Dr. Hanah Nemets and her colleagues at two major institutions in Israel showed significant improvement in depression scores on testing of depressed children who took the supplement compared to those who did not. The example of omega-3 fatty acids demonstrates how many complementary treatments are increasingly subject to research to ensure their safety and value. In the case of herbs and supplements in the United States, the FDA does not regulate these treatments at all so their safety is uncertain, a high degree of variability exists in their quality, and they are often expensive. The more limited research and regulation, and expense of alternative and complementary treatments have not diminished their popularity, nor has it kept highly educated families from using them. Many families recognize that alternative therapies in particular are not as

Treatment

Alternative treatment

The use of non-traditional treatments instead of those typically prescribed in Western medicine. An example would be the use of Chinese herbs to treat depression.

Complementary treatment

The use of non-traditional treatments along with typical treatments prescribed in Western medicine. An example would be the use of yoga with medications for anxiety.

well studied as standard Western medical therapies, but that they have been used for hundreds of years in other cultures. A number of studies looking at the use of alternative medicines have revealed that patients frequently leave their doctors "out of the loop" and use such treatments on the advice of friends and relatives. Studies also revealed that those using these alternative treatments believe them to be safe because they are "natural" or holistic. It is very important to realize that any treatment, natural or otherwise, can have potential risks and side effects, and can even have dangerous interactions if taken with commonly prescribed or over-the-counter medications. On the other hand, some people feel helped by alternative treatments, and it would be a disservice to assume that they offer no benefit to certain patients.

It is very important to realize that any treatment, natural or otherwise, can have potential risks and side effects, and can even have dangerous interactions if taken with commonly prescribed or over-the-counter medications.

If you are reading this book, hopefully you are seeking help from a medical doctor either for primary or psychiatric care. Make a habit of letting your doctor know what other treatments you are providing your child besides the ones she recommends. Your child's health and future really depends on having an open line of communication with your doctor about treatments you are considering. Some doctors may not be familiar with these treatments. In such a case, it is a chance for you and your child's doctor (and other treating clinicians) to work together as a team in a treatment plan. Many doctors appreciate being informed, may be able to tell you about the benefits and possible risks involved with alternative treatments, and are often eager to learn more about other treatments that are of interest to their patients.

Geraldine's comment:

Before we accepted the role of standard psychiatric medications, we tried a variety of alternate therapies—natural remedies, including diets, serotonin enhancers. I've always liked the idea of using natural products—I use them myself and I recommend them to my elderly parents, one of whom is developing Alzheimer's. I discovered some fish oil supplements that to me tasted pretty good, but neither of my kids would take it in the doses recommended. Ultimately, we gave up on those and we arrived at the conclusion that mainstream medication would be more appropriate, at least for Lexie, and it has been to some extent. With children, though, medication is really one part of the larger picture.

80. What is cognitive–behavioral therapy, and how does it work?

Cognitive-behavioral therapy or CBT, as it is better known, is a combined treatment approach using cognitive therapy and behavior therapy. Cognitive therapy focuses on evaluating and correcting distorted beliefs or thinking patterns, while behavior therapy seeks to adapt or change inappropriate types of behavior using different learning strategies. CBT addresses both "thinking" and "doing" in its treatment of various problems. CBT has been applied to a variety of psychiatric disorders, which include depression, suicidality, anxiety, and social skills deficiencies. Many types of CBT exist, with a range of the amount of thinking and doing therapy involved. Older children, such as preteens and teens, can respond to CBT that uses more cognitive (thinking) approaches, while younger, more immature children such as preschoolers and elementary school-aged youngsters respond better to the CBT that uses more behavioral (doing) approaches. CBT can be given in the individual, group, or family-based format. In the individual and group formats, thought processes and skill building are more on the child's level, where the family-based format includes parents' thinking and training as they apply to the child. CBT is considered one of the most successful types of psychotherapy for children with mood disorders and its use may, at times, avoid or minimize the need for medications. The main drawback of CBT is that its availability in the community is often limited and not enough practitioners are comfortable using it (due to the high level of training it requires) in their work with children. Nonetheless, your doctor may be able to help you identify local, qualified CBT practitioners who might be of value in your child's treatment.

The premise of IPT is that interpersonal problems with others lead to depression in the individual. IPT seeks to reduce depressive symptoms and maintain or improve current relationships with valued people in the child's life.

81. What is interpersonal therapy, and how does it help in depression?

Interpersonal therapy (IPT) is a type of time-limited individual psychotherapy, first developed for adults, and more recently, modified for teenagers, that is used to treat depression. The premise of IPT is that interpersonal problems with others lead to depression in the individual. IPT seeks to reduce depressive symptoms and maintain or improve current relationships with valued people in the child's life. Research on talk therapies such as IPT for children and adolescents is still in its early stages; however, several studies on IPT with adolescents (IPT-A) have shown positive results where those who received it had an improvement in depression that lasted well beyond the end of the treatment period.

82. Does group therapy help children with mood disorders?

Group therapy is an approach to treatment that usually involves a small group of similarly aged children or adolescents (usually between 6 and 12 individuals) who are led by 1 or 2 skilled adult mental health professionals in a regular meeting. The group often meets for 45 minutes to an hour, and can involve talking, play, or creative arts to facilitate communication and relationships, develop skills, or increase knowledge among the members. The number of meetings for the group can be limited (e.g., 10 sessions) with the same members, or they can be ongoing and allow open membership over time. Members of a group could have the same diagnosis, such as depression or ADHD, or be of the same gender with similar social needs (e.g., the need to develop better interpersonal skills) or have a common stressful event (e.g., the loss of a parent or major medical illness like cancer). Group therapy can be given in several different settings. A school, clinic, shelter, or private office equipped to accommodate a number of people at once are the most common places where group treatment occurs. A variety of methods and formats exist for group therapy, just as with individual therapy. Some of the types of group therapy include psychoeducational groups, where topics such as maintenance of health and wellness with psychiatric disorders, medications, or basic facts about specific illnesses may be taught and discussed. Groups that focus on processing feelings and developing coping skills include CBT groups and social skills training groups.

Not only children, but parents and other family members can benefit from group therapy directed at relatives of children with psychiatric disorders. Family psycho-educational groups exist to support a child's individual, group, and/or family therapy. Other types of groups include those focused on building skills needed in supporting a child with psychiatric illness.

Group therapy can be quite helpful for children because it makes use of the opinions and experiences of peers, which are especially important for youngsters who may have trouble engaging with adults in treatment. Since children are used to attending school and spending time with other children, the social context of group therapy can seem more "natural" to them than sitting one on one with an adult therapist. A youngster may often feel alone and isolated in her struggles with psychiatric illness, and group treatment with others who have similar problems can make that experience more tolerable.

Group therapy can be very valuable indeed in the treatment of children with mood disorders. Some examples of groups that have been shown to be beneficial for children and teens include CBT group therapy to address depressive and suicidal symptoms. With bipolar and other mood disorders, a highly structured type of family psychoeducational group treatment, known as multifamily psychoeducation groups, created by researchers at The Ohio State University, seems to be a promising treatment option for families afflicted with these illnesses.

Unfortunately, group treatment for children is not as readily available as individual treatment. There are a variety of reasons which account for the scarcity, including geographic shortages of trained mental health professionals, lack of space or opportunity among private practitioners to hold such groups, and lack of training among available clinicians. Despite the limited availability of group therapy, it remains worthwhile to explore with your doctor if group treatment is an appropriate option for your child and family.

83. Are there any other treatments besides medications and "talk therapy" mentioned here that are available to children and families?

In addition to CBT, IPT, group, and family therapies described, other therapies are available to children. These include individual **psychodynamic psychotherapy**, play therapy, and various other therapies using the creative arts such as fine art, music, dance, or drama. Psychodynamic psychotherapy encompasses the theories and techniques of many important thinkers in the field, which includes psychoanalysis. Sigmund Freud first developed psychoanalysis as an intense form of evaluation and treatment (meeting several times a week) where the therapist and patient work together to identify and resolve conflicts that occurred in the patient's early childhood by bringing them into present awareness and effecting changes in current behavior and emotional life.

Psychodynamic psychotherapy can be very useful in the treatment of youth with depressive, anxious, or bipolar disorders. It focuses on the mind, including conscious and unconscious elements that make up our inner lives. Patients who are reflective and verbally oriented may find this style of treatment especially beneficial. The psychiatrist, Glen Gabbard, and other prominent thinkers in the field make a number of observations about the utility of psychodynamic psychotherapy in patients. For

Psychodynamic psychotherapy

An intense type of therapy that focuses on the mind as the source of human feelings, thoughts, and behaviors. It is usually a verbal therapy in more mature individuals, but in younger children and adolescents, it can also be achieved through play.

143

example, psychodynamic psychotherapy can help youngsters with bipolar disorder get help in making connections with, and better understanding of, the extremes of their illness, when they are both unwell (manic) and well. Because it heightens peoples' awareness of the personal meanings of things, this type of therapy is valuable in helping patients manage stress, reduce relapses, and understanding the impact of the illness on their life as well as their families' lives. It may be helpful in achieving the important commitment of taking medications to control mania, and in the case of ambivalence or noncompliance with medications, it may be helpful in allowing the patient to understand the reasons for these feelings. Over time, a relationship with a doctor or other therapist specializing in psychodynamic psychotherapy can help a young person bridge important developmental transitions and the weather the "ups and downs" of having bipolar disorder.

As mentioned, psychodynamic psychotherapy can occur through conversations between therapists and patients, but it can also occur through play. **Play therapy** includes a range of therapeutic approaches with children using toys or props. Some types of play therapy are formal, organized, and based on various theories of psychodynamic psychotherapy, while others are more informal and less structured. Play therapy is especially important in working with younger children because it does not rely on a high level of verbal skill as do some of the other styles of psychotherapy commonly used in adults. Most professionals consider play for children the equivalent of "work" for adults. Play is their way of mastering skills in the world that include completing tasks, processing ideas, solving problems, and developing relationships needed for their growth and development, and also feeling safe. Adults sometimes have trouble appreciating the value of play in the

Play therapy

Includes a range of therapeutic approaches using toys or props. Play is children's way of mastering things in the world that include completing tasks, processing ideas, solving problems, and developing relationships needed for their growth and development, and also feeling safe.

lives of children, from both a recreational and therapeutic standpoint. They might see their child's job as "going to school" and "listening to one's parents." However, without play, those other tasks of school and fulfilling a role as a family member are really quite meaningless for a child's well-being. It is almost certain that some type of play therapy is included in the work being done with your child, especially if she is a young child. Some professionals, who are highly trained in the technical aspects of play, may have the title "play therapist." Others may not have such formal qualification but are, nonetheless, experienced enough to use play in their treatment. Perhaps you are fully aware of the play that goes on during your child's sessions with the therapist, as your child talks about it later with you. It may seem silly and meaningless. You should probably realize that your daughter may not be able to talk with another adult about various problems that she is experiencing, but may easily be able to communicate about them through play. For those parents who want a more active role in the treatment, some play therapists are able to include the parent in treatment, depending on the situation and the techniques being practiced.

Other therapies using the creative arts are frequently used with children for the same reasons as play therapy with toys, as they draw upon a child's nonverbal means of communication and expression, and can be quite powerful in helping those who are suffering from a variety of psychiatric disorders, including those who have speech and language problems, autism, brain injuries, or mental retardation in addition to mood disorders. Often, these methods will be part of a larger repertoire of approaches used in treating your child's emotional problems, and may complement other treatments such as medications and family therapy.

Most likely, your child's doctor will be able to help you develop an appropriate treatment plan and decide what types of therapeutic modalities are indicated for her. The AACAP Facts for Families series succinctly describes the different options for psychotherapy in children (see Question 100 for further details).

Geraldine's comment:
I can't overemphasize the importance of play for young children. It really helps adults work with children on their level. I recall a consultation with one child mental health professional—there were no toys in the waiting room or office! Needless to say, it revealed a lot about his approach to children and lack of effort to bring them into things.

84. When should we go to an emergency room or seek hospitalization?

Ideally, crises in a family struggling with a child's mood disorder are best handled in session with your treating doctor. Emergency rooms (ERs) and hospitals, while they are incredibly important resources in the community, can offer only temporary solutions at best. Your doctor should be alerted right away in the event of a serious situation with your child, and guidance about whether to seek an ER or hospital visit should be sought as well.

In general, violent and dangerous behavior such as aggression in the home, assault toward family members, or the immediate threat of violence, are some situations where the use of an ER is indicated, usually by calling 911 and getting police and ambulance assistance. Suicidal behaviors, such as an attempt or an imminent threat by overdose, injury, or weapon, are other examples that warrant attention in an ER. A hospital stay is usually advised if the child's safety in the home continues to be in question beyond an ER stay. After many hours or a night in the ER, many youngsters are able to "pull themselves together" and behave in a way that is far more appropriate and are able to go home. Ultimately, the ER doctor will make the determination if it is wise to return home. A parent may be frustrated by the discharge of her child from the ER after an incident of inappropriate behavior occurs, but should continue to work with her child's primary treating doctor to prevent future such behavior.

If the ER, in conjunction with your child's doctor, decides that hospitalization is needed, it would usually be for a few days or weeks. The goals of hospitalization are to establish a safe, highly supervised environment to monitor your child and help her get back on track. The hospital stay may be a place for medications to be monitored more carefully, or changes in her medication regimen to be made that were difficult to achieve under parental supervision. For a teenager who is abusing drugs in addition to suffering from emotional problems, the hospital can serve as a place where the illegal substances are removed, and can offer the child a chance to be treated for underlying problems that are frequently masked by the effects of drugs and alcohol. The hospital is also a more structured setting than home, and may lend itself to helping your child get back into appropriate routines that are needed to function in the community. The hospital is usually a restrictive environment where a child is removed from the usual influences in the community (such as friends and family) and can serve a temporary function in helping the child focus on her problems more effectively. An inpatient psychiatric unit frequently also has intensive treatment sessions such as groups and individual therapy that may also prove useful to your child. Overall, however, a hospital stay is a short-term treatment option in your child's experience with a mood

For a teenager who is abusing drugs in addition to suffering from emotional problems, the hospital can serve as a place where the illegal substances are removed, and can offer the child a chance to be treated for underlying problems that are frequently masked by the effects of drugs and alcohol.

Treatment

disorder. Hospitalization almost never addresses the stressors or ongoing conflicts that predispose your child to the undesirable behaviors that got them there in the first place. Those issues are generally chronic in nature and best addressed in the outpatient setting with your doctor and other treating professionals.

85. Once depression is treated, is it cured?

Nothing is as much of a relief and cause for hope as knowing that your child's illness is successfully treated, and you can all go on with your life as before. Unfortunately, many illnesses recur, and depression is among them. Studies have shown that major depressive disorder in children and adolescents recurs 40% of the time in 2 years, and 70% of the time in 5 years. Other types of depressive illnesses, such as dysthymia and the depressive component of bipolar disorder, also frequently experience recurrences. These are concerning figures, but are likely due to complicating factors. These numbers tell us little about risk factors for recurrence, such as ongoing stressors or strong family history of depression. Furthermore, it is hard to know if the first episode of depression is part of a larger pattern of recurrences that are going to happen over a lifetime, or if it is the first presentation of a bipolar illness.

It may feel discouraging to know that recurrence of depression is so common. However, maintaining treatment for periods of time beyond the initial remission of the episode can help delay or possibly prevent the recurrences. **Remission** is defined as substantial reduction or complete resolution of depressive symptoms between 2 weeks and 2 months. A relapse is defined as the presentation of depressive symptoms within this

Remission

Reduction or resolution of depressive symptoms in the early stages of the illness, between 2 weeks and 2 months.

period of 2 weeks and 2 months. A recurrence is defined as the presentation of a new episode depression beyond 2 months after remission has been achieved. As mentioned previously, experts recommend treatment of depression for at least 6–12 months after remission of the first episode. Treatment includes the use of medicine and/or psychotherapy, depending on what is advised by your doctor. In addition, addressing other risk factors such as a highly conflicted family situation or parent-child relationship through treatment may further reduce your child's chances of a relapse or recurrence. Maintaining a healthy lifestyle in your child, especially with regard to enough sleep and appropriate diet and activity level, may also reduce the risk factors for another episode of depression or mania.

86. I know someone whose son with bipolar disorder killed himself. What went wrong? Didn't anyone realize he needed help?

Suicide is the third leading cause of death in youth between the ages of 15 and 24, according to the Centers for Disease Control and Prevention. The AACAP reports that some 2,000 teenagers commit suicide every year in the United States. The reasons for an adolescent to kill himself stem from the inability to handle various situations such as stressful life events, family or school problems, or a failed romance. Males comprise the overwhelming majority of completed suicide in young people. Many factors beyond age and sex influence who will commit suicide. Mental illness, such as bipolar disorder, and concurrent abuse of drugs or alcohol increases the risk of suicide in youth considerably. Also, a history of prior suicide attempts (especially a male), and/or a family history of a relative who committed suicide, puts a child or adolescent at higher risk for eventually killing himself. The presence of a gun in the home increases the risk of suicide by five times, according to the AAP.

If your friend's son was already diagnosed with bipolar disorder and sought any help, he was already in the minority of people who kill themselves, as the majority of those who take their own life don't seek help at all. Even if a suicidal person in under treatment, it can be challenging to control the harmful feelings. Sadly, many youngsters with bipolar disorder kill themselves while experiencing the extremes of mania, depression, anxiety, and/or drug intoxication. Often, these individuals feel lonely and estranged from their family and friends. At times, others in the life of a suicidal person may not be aware of the degree of suffering experienced before a suicide occurs.

Without knowing the circumstances of your friend's son or his illness, it's hard to make any conclusions about what led to the suicide. What you can do for your friend now is ensure that she has support and guidance from others in grieving her terrible loss. If you are concerned about your own child's risk for suicide, your doctor should be able to help you evaluate the situation and serve as an important resource for information and recommendations.

87. What can I do to make it safer for my teenager who feels suicidal?

The reader is referred to the AACAP Facts for Families handout as well as the AAP handout on suicide (see Question 100 for links) where detailed information on suicide and measures to prevent it are given.

At times, the doctor and family might agree to continue to work with a teenager who feels suicidal without hospitalizing him. Managing a suicidal teen in the community can be done successfully, but it can also be highly stressful and requires careful attention at the level of home and family. First, the family should remove all firearms and lethal medications from the home. Without access to a gun in particular, the chances of committing suicide are reduced considerably. Both the AAP and AACAP advise that an alternate, but less desirable option to removing firearms is to secure them in a locked cabinet, preferably in an undisclosed location in the home. Potentially fatal medication when overdosed (such as tricyclic antidepressants) should not be kept in the home of a suicidal person at all. It may be difficult to completely "suicide-proof" the home since common dangerous objects such as knives, various over-the-counter medications, and household solvents can't be eliminated in most homes; motivated or impulsive teenagers are somehow able to find less obvious ways to harm themselves using things from around the house. However, the family should make its best effort to "clean out the place" of weapons and dangerous materials.

If the use of drugs and/or alcohol is complicating your teen's illness, then that needs to be addressed aggressively, as substance use will worsen suicidal behavior. Underage drinking in the home might be eliminated by removing alcohol from the liquor cabinets, as well as by providing a high level of adult supervision at home. Other opportunities for a teenager to access drugs or alcohol outside of home can be reduced by placing strict limits on your child's access to money and knowing your child's peer group and social circles. Treatment for substance abuse should receive high priority in the care of a youngster with a mood disorder who experiences suicidality.

If the use of drugs and/or alcohol is complicating your teen's illness, then that needs to be addressed aggressively, as substance use will worsen suicidal behavior.

151

In general, a suicidal teenager needs to be highly supervised by adults, and avoid being left at home alone or unescorted to and from school. A responsible and supportive family member or trusted adult should be around to at least provide companionship, if not supervision, and should be able to act immediately if an emergency situation arises.

Finally, close monitoring by your teenager's doctor will be necessary. This could mean more frequent appointments, telephone calls, and possibly visiting the emergency room. At times, your doctor or emergency room doctor may feel psychiatric hospitalization is indicated to further ensure your son's supervision and safety.

As parents, you are often the first to perceive a downturn in your child's mental health, which may include suicidality. Observable signs of impending suicide may include an increase in hopelessness or negativistic thinking, further withdrawal from family or friends, or attempts to have closure or finality on aspects of the child's life. Nothing, however, substitutes for being direct and asking a youngster specific questions about suicidal thoughts or plans, and communicating that information to the treating doctor. **Remember, asking about suicide does not make it more likely to happen**. Professional experience has shown this to be true, and there is no scientific evidence to support otherwise. An open dialogue with your teenager about the topic of suicide may be able to clarify the degree of suicidal thinking present, and guide you and your doctor as to how to best keep her safe.

Remember, asking about suicide does not make it more likely to happen.

PART FIVE

Surviving

What should we tell teachers about our son's
medications?

We recently discovered that our daughter has been
hiding her medications instead of taking them for
the last 2 months. What can we do?

My wife and I disagree about the treatment for
our daughter's bipolar illness. Is this a problem?

More . . .

88. I feel guilty that my child has become depressed. My daughter blames me for it. What can I do now?

Parental guilt is common when a child becomes ill. Parents struggle to understand what, if anything, they did that contributed to their child's disorder. Sometimes the things that a parent may feel caused the depression are logical, but sometimes they're not. It's easy to believe that parenting style and other aspects of a child's upbringing are the sole causes of a mental disorder, but usually illnesses have multiple, complicated etiologies which include a child's individual coping skills, biological predisposition to neurochemical events, and life stressors. Many of these factors may have been out of the parents' control but cause guilt anyway because a mother or father would have wanted to be able to protect the child from their negative effects.

You probably feel badly enough about your daughter's condition as it is, but being blamed for it by her is probably making matters worse. It may make you feel sad, or even angry, to be targeted as a source for the illness that appears to have happened despite all your best efforts to prevent it. You may be puzzled to hear that it is your fault, since your experience of your daughter's life leading up to the depression may be far different than her experience. You might feel your daughter caused her own problems and now blames you for what she should admit to herself. Perhaps you think she is being ungrateful in failing to recognize all that you have done and continue to do to help her.

That having been said, there may be things you, as the parent, can do to help improve the situation. Improving the patterns of communication between you and your child often helps considerably. This may require hard work as a family in treatment, especially since parent-child communication style goes back many years and habits which don't work well may be hard to break. Professional guidance from your doctor and/or other therapists will help you observe and understand what actions positively and negatively affect your relationship. With that knowledge, you may then be able to change some of those actions. Remember, part of being depressed can include having a negative view on everything, including those you love. Depression rarely happens from one cause, and the inability to explain its origin may lead a teenager to blame those who are closest to her. Your daughter may already have trouble saying what's on her mind, but the added complication of depression can make that even more difficult. Even at her worst, your daughter really does need you to help her get through the depression. She may be able to express that when she is doing a bit better and that may be a time to address the fact that her words can hurt you too.

One thing that you may want to do is talk with other parents who are going through the same things you are. Patient and family advocacy groups such as NAMI, and the Depression and Bipolar Support Alliance (DBSA) (see Question 100) often provide opportunities for parents to hear about experiences like theirs, share resources and wisdom, and lend their ears. It can be a tremendous help to know that others are in your situation, too. Other parents can be a wealth of information, suggestions, and empathy during this difficult time for you.

89. I am embarrassed that my son needs to see a psychiatrist. Should I keep it a secret from others in our community?

Mental illness is considered a stigma in many cultures, even ours, despite the fact that so much is known about it, treatment for it is so readily available, and so many advocacy groups exist for it. Not long ago, the U.S. Surgeon General declared that reducing the stigma of mental illness in children is a national priority. Your community's openness to mental illness can influence how you feel about having a psychiatric diagnosis in a family member. It can also weigh upon your willingness to talk freely with others about the illness. As a parent, however, you need to be able to balance your relationship with the outside world with the one you have with your child. Whatever sense of shame you feel about your child's illness may affect your child's attitude toward his illness, and his self-esteem. Your child may believe that you are embarrassed of *him* and that perhaps *he* is a bad person for having the illness. The shared embarrassment can have a demoralizing and negative effect on the family as well as the individual and create a more difficult path to recovery from the illness. The energy required to keep secrets about your child's health can also produce considerable stress for both you and your child. You may spend more time worrying about what people may find out or think, rather than focusing on helping your child and family get through the illness and get on with life.

As the parent of a youngster with a psychiatric disorder, you are actually in a position of being able to educate others about it and help foster a frank and nonjudgmental approach in dealing with the problem. The most effective means of destigmatizing mental illness is to talk about it in straightforward terms, and treat it like any other chronic, medical condition. You might be surprised to see that your friends and family may not react as poorly to such discussion as you had feared, and they may even be source of support to you during an otherwise tough time. It may also open up opportunities for others to talk about their own emotional health and problems without feeling judged.

Examining your own personal concerns about having to see a psychiatrist may help you to overcome shame about it. Are you worried that it reflects badly on you as a parent because you couldn't help your child yourself and need to go to a professional? Do you think people will ridicule you or your child for having a mental illness? Have you or another family member had a previous bad experience with mental illness that leads you to keep quiet about this one? Does your extended family judge you constantly, and would this serve as just another area where you will feel criticized? These questions and others are appropriate concerns to bring to your doctor, who may have further thoughts and recommendations on how best to handle the situation.

Examining your own personal concerns about having to see a psychiatrist may help you to overcome shame about it.

Geraldine's comment:

It was our experience that while our relatives were generally supportive of what we wanted to do for our children, they weren't able to offer much either. The grandparents felt helpless and an elderly great aunt and others just wanted solutions when they heard about particular problems, which we obviously couldn't provide. It was also hard as the parents because nobody [among the relatives] believes how hard it is day to day, since the kids appear so well to them whenever they visit.

157

90. *What should we tell his teachers about our son's medications?*

Not all teachers need to know about a child's medications. What you choose to share with your son's teacher(s) is up to you. However, it can be very helpful for parents to keep their child's teacher informed about certain medications, especially if he is still in elementary school and has one teacher for most of his classes. If your son is on a medicine for ADHD that is intended to help with concentration, staying on task, or in his seat for example, the teacher will be able to observe and let you know if it is helping achieve those goals. If he is on an SSRI for depression or anxiety and it has some side effects such as feeling sleepy, the teacher will be able to let you know if he is falling asleep in class. You can bring this information back to your doctor and discuss whether the time of administration can be changed to improve wakefulness during the day. Sometimes it's helpful to alert guidance counselors about your child's medication, if your son is seen often outside of the classroom during the week. Guidance counselors can also be helpful in providing feedback about your son's response to a new medication.

Some medicines that are given several times a day may need to be given at school by someone qualified to dispense them, such as a nurse. In these cases, it may be helpful for the teacher and other school personnel to be made aware of the need for medication dosing during the day.

91. I became severely depressed after the birth of my daughter. What effect will this have on my baby now, and as she grows up?

After giving birth, postpartum depression is an occasional, but very serious, complication. It is a more severe and extreme disturbance in the mother that occurs aside from the more common "postpartum blues" which present as moodiness and irritability due to shifting hormone levels after giving birth. A mother suffering from untreated postpartum depression can exhibit behaviors that can be harmful not only for herself, but also to her baby. A depressed new mother may not be able to participate in the demanding care of her newborn, especially the round-the-clock feeding and nurturing that is required. Newborns of depressed mothers can exhibit poor weight gain and have problems forming the appropriate bonds with their mothers, and possibly other people. Such babies may be neglected by their mothers and fail to receive the emotional support needed early in their lives, and experience developmental delays such as walking and talking later than normal. In more extreme situations, a depressed mother may resort to violent acts, such as suicide or even infanticide. Even if you suffer from depression that you feel is not that severe, over time, this can have a negative effect on a growing child. Babies are not the only ones who suffer when the mother is depressed; a depressed mother who goes untreated can have a serious, negative impact on children of all ages. Children of depressed mothers often internalize their mothers' depressive symptoms and outlook on life, and later may suffer from depression themselves. You may not realize that your ability to be a caring and loving parent is severely compromised by untreated depression. Depressed parents, especially mothers, are frequently observed to be more irritable, impatient, and harsh toward their children. Even with this knowledge, it can be hard for a mother to seek help. Mothers frequently neglect caring for themselves in favor of the needs of the family, feeling they don't have enough time or energy. However, a mother cannot take good care of her children if she is not well herself. The reasons for a parent, especially a mother, to seek treatment for her own depression (or any other mental illness, for that matter) are very compelling, since they extend far beyond the woman herself.

The example of postpartum depression is an important one, as it also speaks for the problem of families with one or more parents with a mood disorder or any serious emotional disturbance. Without proper treatment, these parents' experiences can have a severe, negative impact on the upbringing of their children. Children in such families are at much higher risk for becoming ill themselves and can present with psychiatric illnesses at a younger age, and perhaps have more severe symptoms as a result of having an ill parent. This unfortunate scenario could, over time, lead to those children becoming impaired adults and allow the suffering to continue for the next generation.

Geraldine's comment:
Even though I didn't experience depression during pregnancy, I feel my experience as an expectant mother really impacted upon our daughter. I was under the most stress imaginable during my pregnancy. The high level of stress hormones, the lifestyle...the result is that our daughter is neither my husband nor me. She's very different. How much was biological and how

much was environmental? There's a lot of guilt associated with that as a parent. It's easy feel the blame for what happened, especially as a mother.

92. My friend's daughter is terminally ill from a brain tumor, and appears depressed. What's the point of treating her depression?

A major illness, such as cancer, is generally a cause for a serious emotional reaction. In fact, adjustment disorders, as previously discussed, are rather common with a serious medical diagnosis, especially in the early stages of diagnosis and treatment. Symptoms of diagnosable depression can occur in reaction to the damaging effects of the treatments themselves—brain and other organ dysfunction, delayed appearance of puberty, loss of future fertility, disfiguration, numerous painful procedures, or poorly controlled pain, to name only a few causes. The symptoms of poor appetite and loss of pleasure in activities are fairly common among cancer patients. Many other causes for depression have been described among pediatric cancer patients. The illness usually is considered terminal after a period of failed treatments. Not only does the child feel depressed as a result of such misfortune, but family members may as well.

The hopelessness of the situation at end-stage, however, should not determine that depression go untreated. In the community of cancer professionals, it is considered increasingly important that a child should have a reasonable quality of life during cancer treatment and, if terminal, also during the later stages of her life. A comfortable and peaceful existence for the child at the end of her life is desirable, not only for the child but

In the community of cancer professionals, it is considered increasingly important that a child should have a reasonable quality of life during cancer treatment and, if terminal, also during the later stages of her life.

Surviving

also for her family who will be surviving her loss. A depressed child may not be able to experience such comfort without being treated for the depression. Your friend deserves to know that her daughter was given the best possible care in all regards, both physically and emotionally. This knowledge can be helpful in her own bereavement process.

93. We recently discovered that our daughter has been hiding her medications instead of taking them for the last 2 months. What can we do?

A recurring theme throughout this book is that older children, especially teenagers, have mixed feelings about psychiatric treatment in general, especially medications. Many adolescents stop taking their medications during the course of their treatment. They may dislike the idea of taking a substance that will interfere with or control their body. They may not like the side effects such as sedation, weight gain, or acne. They might not agree with their parents about taking it in the first place, but pretend to do so in order to keep the peace at home. They might feel no effect whatsoever from the medication and, therefore, assume taking them is a waste of time. On the other hand, teenagers may feel better after taking medications, assume that they are "cured" of their illness, and decide that they no longer need the medicines to keep them well. Whatever the reason for covertly stopping the medication, it must be addressed and you should try to find out from your daughter why she was playing this charade. Sometimes, you may be able to overcome the problem, such as by modifying a side effect: a sedating medication might be taken later in the day in order keep her more alert in school or a change from one medicine to another to limit weight gain might be possible. Another example might include a visit to the dermatologist to help improve acne made worse by lithium. Progress can occur if you can help address the side effect problem and at least obtain an agreement to take the medicine. The presence of some medications can be tested for in the blood (e.g., lithium or valproate level), so monitoring would be another way of knowing if the medication is being taken properly. Some medicines, though not all, are available in forms other than traditional tablets and capsules that must be swallowed. These include liquid preparations, rapidly dissolving tablets, skin patches, and occasionally, injections. These other delivery methods may improve **compliance** (cooperation or, in this case, the ability to take the medications as directed). A discussion with your doctor about such alternatives might reveal options to consider for your child.

Even an adult would feel discouraged if she could not tolerate the side effect profile of a particular medication regimen. Again, it's always a good idea to supervise the taking of medicine, even for a teenager, at least as far as swallowing the pills. It may seem extreme to stand there while she takes the pill and ask to check her mouth afterward, but if she has lost your trust in taking it responsibly on her own, you may need to do this, at least temporarily, until she regains your trust. As mentioned earlier, one thing you should not do is give the medicine secretly by hiding it in her food or drink. This method is no less deceptive than her pretending to take the medicine, and just reinforces the

Surviving

Compliance

The extent to which treatment recommendations are followed by a patient.

sense that trust can't be maintained in your home, among adults or children.

You may find yourself at an impasse if your daughter refuses outright to the take the medicine. If so, you may be able to use withholding of privileges or restrictions to help persuade her to make a better choice. Discuss this matter with your child and your psychiatrist, and perhaps you can come up with some solutions together. If your doctor feels strongly about it and it is a serious enough matter, hospitalization may be an option to ensure compliance, but that route is usually reserved for dangerous behavior. Furthermore, the hospital only works in the short term, while the child is in the more restrictive environment. It does not guarantee that once back home she will not fall back into her previous habits. Sometimes the alternative of being in a hospital or other restrictive setting is enough to motivate a teenager to take her medicine. Bear in mind that if you use hospitalization as a bargaining tool to encourage cooperation, you should not back down and must follow through if necessary. Empty talk will only send the message that you don't really mean what you say, and you probably won't be taken seriously in the future with regard to this matter.

94. I recently discovered that my teenager has been skipping his appointments for psychotherapy. How can I deal with this?

Skipped appointments usually imply that a person is ambivalent about or rejecting the treatment. It could reflect your son's anger at you for requiring the treatment, his refusal to acknowledge the problem for which you are arranging the appointments, or some concern about the therapy he is not voicing. Your son may want you to believe he is attending therapy rather than telling you outright that he will not go, as the former might satisfy you in the short run and avoid further conflict with you. Adolescents are constantly struggling to assert their independence and, like cutting class or skipping school, they may do the same with their appointments. Understandably, this can be infuriating to the parent who may be spending a lot of hard-earned money or sacrificing time from a busy schedule to make arrangements or even participate themselves in the treatment. A teenager may have limited appreciation for this reality, just as he does when he loses an expensive pair of sneakers or jewelry and demands a replacement without much thought. It is a hard task to teach an adolescent about time and money.

Maybe you're upset that the doctor or therapist did not inform you right away about the absences. It's a complicated position for someone treating your teenager to act both on his behalf and as his "probation officer." Some clinicians will alert the parents about missed appointments, but others may not, as they could feel the child's actions are part of the treatment process. Teenagers easily lose trust in adults whom they think are agents of their parents and further withdraw from therapy. As a parent, you may also be troubled about being charged for missed appointments, or feel excluded from the treatment process. Having a frank discussion with your child's clinician about your feelings is the most useful way to approach this type of situation.

It is crucial to find out why this is happening before you can do something to turn it around. Sometimes it's hard to get a straight answer from a teenager as to why he did something that you find wrong. Your son's doctor may have some suggestions and may choose to incorporate this struggle around appointments into the treatment. Some things are easier to fix, such as an inconvenient time (too early in the morning before school, when a teen is likely to oversleep), or a time that is in competition with a favorite activity (e.g., sports practice). You, as the parent, need to try to control your frustration around the matter, at least in front of your son, as a strong reaction on your part may actually further fuel his actions if a long-standing pattern of conflict exists between you. Perhaps you are in a position to escort your son to the appointments yourself or arrange for a responsible adult to help him with that until it is clear that he will continue appropriately on his own. If that is not an option, you may have to find an incentive for your son to responsibly attend his appointments or impose a penalty for skipping them, such as granting or withholding his allowance or other privilege.

Even if your son feels that the appointments are not worth his time, it would be a good idea to have him keep going on a regular basis, since the treatment will never gain any momentum if it is too sporadic and infrequent. (It's like exercising—if you do it only once in a while, you will not feel the motivation or benefit of doing it regularly). Also, you may want to know what else he is doing with his time during, or just before, that appointment—is he going home to take a nap because he is too tired all the time, or going out with his friends to smoke marijuana? Solving this type problem is sometimes rather difficult and his reasons for skipping out may all be part of the symptoms of his ailment, like hopelessness or forgetfulness. In this regard, working together with your doctor to address this problem is especially important.

95. My teenaged son is the one with depression. Why do I need to go to some of his appointments? Can't he deal with it on his own?

Even though your teenager has a mind and body of his own and can do most things by himself, he still needs his parents. The relationship with your child is life-long, and especially during tough times, it will be put to the test. An adolescent may tell his mother or father to "go away" or avoid them altogether, but what his parents do or think still matters a great deal to most teenagers. Furthermore a child, no matter what age, is a part of a "system"—your family. What different members think and do within that system will have an impact on each other. Also, by being there for your child, you are giving him the message that even if you don't agree with him all the time, you still support him and want to be part of the solution and not the problem. As a parent, you probably learned long ago that good parenting goes way beyond giving your child the material things he needs (like paying for his treatment). Ask your doctor and your child how much involvement you should have in the treatment, and be available to participate to the extent that is needed.

96. My wife and I disagree about the treatment for our daughter's bipolar illness. Is this a problem?

It is definitely *a problem when parents don't agree on what is best for their child.*

It is *definitely* a problem when parents don't agree on what is best for their child. Since your child was a baby, she has picked up on what Mommy and Daddy think about different things. At times, that was okay and she learned that her mother and father were just two different people with different opinions. However, differing opinions can be confusing to a child and give her a mixed message about what is right or wrong, even if both parents are "right." Sometimes it also puts her in the middle of something that should not be her concern, namely a disagreement between the adults.

If you and your spouse are together in a committed relationship, it is helpful to do what you can to come to an agreement about your daughter's treatment, whether it is a compromise or one opinion over the other. Even if you are separated or divorced, if you are both involved in your daughter's life it is crucial to put your own feelings aside and still try to see eye to eye on what is best for her, showing a "united front" in the matter. If not, she will likely be ambivalent about whatever treatment is being chosen for her and this may cause the treatment to fail. Many parents, unfortunately, are not able to come to agreement on what they want for the child. Regardless, it will be important to tell your doctor that such a conflict exists. This difference of opinion must be taken into consideration, and perhaps even included as part of the treatment in the family work for the child.

Geraldine's comment:

It's a big problem [when a husband and wife dis-agree] because we need to be on the same page in terms of recognizing that our child has a disorder. It was a couple of years of denial back and forth between the two of us. My husband just left it all up to me... [arranging the evaluations, the appointments, the treatments]. He was probably more in denial than I was, being a numbers person [he had more trouble relating to emotional problems]. It was pretty taxing for me to bear the weight of it all on my shoulders.

97. Why does the doctor think we need family therapy? Is he blaming us for causing our daughter's depression?

Family therapy is one part of a larger treatment plan for a youngster with a mood disorder. A child does not live in a vacuum; the actions and opinions of, and relation-ships with other members of the family, especially the parents, are critical determinants of success or failure in treatment. As mentioned earlier, feeling guilt is a com-mon experience of parents with a troubled child. It may be easy to feel blamed for your child's ailment. Bear in mind, however, that rarely does a simple cause and effect theory explain why one child became ill. What may happen in the course of family therapy is that your therapist will make you more aware of patterns of behavior or communication within the family that are demoralizing or counterproductive to your child's emo-tional health. Family therapy comes in several varieties, but regardless of type, it serves to help identify ways of interacting within the family that are more nurturing and healing to the child and his family. Consider the suggestion of family therapy as an opportunity to take a more active role in your child's treatment, rather than as a criticism.

Geraldine's comment:

While I can certainly understand the need for family therapy, I do know what it's like to feel blamed or judged by the professionals evaluating Lexie. One of her school reports made mention of my being late to the evaluation. I would have appreciated it if they would have kept me out of it, or at least discussed their concerns with me rather than put it in writing, which looks more accusatory. I know it's hard not to take things too personally in all this.

98. I am having trouble remembering to give my child his medications. What can I do to help myself do a better job?

Grown-ups have difficulty taking their own medications according to a schedule, so it is no surprise that they might forget their children's pills as well. It is helpful to have an organized pill box for your child with enough chambers for each day to hold a week or more of medicines. This is especially important if a child has more than one pill to take daily. Keep the box in a place that is highly visible and preferably located where routine activities like meals will occur. As a reminder for yourself you could put the box out in the kitchen area the night before and set up breakfast bowls or glasses together, so that taking the pill(s) will be associated with the morning meal. Of course, some children (and parents) skip breakfast, which is generally not a healthy habit, as nearly all psychiatric medications are better taken with or after a meal. Try to make breakfast a daily ritual and other things like taking medication in the morning can be easier as well.

Having the pill box associated with other activities in the day, like the afternoon snack, dinner, or brushing teeth before bedtime is also helpful.

Your son or daughter can help you in the process of daily pill administration. If she is old enough to remember, she can get credit for reminding you that it is time for the medicine in the form or points or tokens as part of a behavior plan that will yield some rewards (prizes, allowance, or privileges) at the end of the week. She can also earn points for taking the medicine properly if that is a struggle. A written schedule can help families keep track of several medications in a day's time. A child can help make the schedule as part of taking responsibility for her health. Posting the schedule on the refrigerator or bulletin board (if you have one) can help, too. Talk further with your doctor about what arrangement will work best for you.

99. I can no longer afford to pay for my child's treatment as it is too expensive. What options to I have?

Unlike pediatric and other medical care, quality mental health care in the United States can be very costly, even for the insured:

Geraldine's comment:
All said and done, it took thousands of dollars for us to get all the evaluations done on our children. People pay $5,000 each for the neuropsychological testing which is not deductible. At one point, I even took my daughter to a big name expert in the field. Again, it cost several thousand dollars. In retrospect, it felt like a real waste, since she's still suffering, but

we remain determined to get the right treatment. At some stage in the future, we might have to worry if we can afford to keep their assessments and treatments going at this rate.

There are several reasons for this unfortunate reality. Private health insurance plans often limit the frequency and reimbursement for mental health visits, leading to fewer psychiatrists and other professionals on insurance panels. This inequity is being fought across the country through political efforts influencing public policy for "Mental Health Parity." Furthermore, treatment for psychiatric disorders may require weekly visits, far more often than a child may go to her pediatrician in a few months' time. In some parts of the country, families pay out of pocket for their children's psychiatric therapy. Working families may qualify for public health insurance which could make access to therapy a bit easier, but often they find they are ineligible. Aside from seeing a private psychiatrist, most large medical centers have outpatient psychiatric clinics where public insurance is accepted or, if uninsured, a family may pay the fees on a "sliding scale" based on their income. If a family cannot afford all the medication expenses, most major pharmaceutical companies have patient assistance programs where the medicines can be obtained at little or no cost, provided you are able to submit proof of your financial situation. Your doctor may be able to recommend a less expensive alternative to a costly medication, if available, such as a generic versus brand name product and prescribe it. Your doctor may also have further suggestions on cost containment measures in your child's treatment.

If a family cannot afford all the medication expenses, most major pharmaceutical companies have patient assistance programs where the medicines can be obtained at little or no cost. . . .

100. Where can I find more information on childhood depression and bipolar disorder?

Hopefully this book has answered some important questions you may have about childhood mood disorders. I recommend the following resources on the Internet, as well as organizations and books to help you in your continued understanding and management of the different challenges associated with depression and bipolar disorder in children. I also hope you will find them useful in helping your child achieve a healthy and productive life.

Healthy Lifestyle and Weight Management Links:

www.nhlbi.nih.gov/health/public/heart/obesity/wecan/whats-we-can/

National Heart Lung and Blood Institute's (NHLBI) educational program for parents and children on maintaining a healthy weight

www.nhlbi.nih.gov/health/public/sleep/starslp/funpad.pdf

A coloring book available through the NHLBI for children, educating about healthy sleep habits

www.nhlbi.nih.gov/health/public/sleep/starslp/teachers/sleep_diary.htm

A sleep diary made by the NHLBI for families to use with their doctor to record times during the week when a child gets up in the morning, goes to bed at night, and how he/she was feeling each day

Surviving

www.mypyramid.gov/kids/index.html

The United States Department of Agriculture's website that helps children use the "food pyramid" to make healthy choices in diet and lifestyle

www.cdc.gov/nccdphp/dnpa/nutrition/nutrition_for_ everyone/healthy_weight/

Department of Health and Human Services (HHS) Centers for Disease Control (CDC) and Prevention website link for nutrition and weight management

www.calolive.org/images/download/pdf/edu_ggg_diary. pdf

An excellent blank food diary for children prepared by the California Olive Industry

www.bam.gov

The CDC website for children to use presenting information on various health related topics including diet, exercise, safety, and prevention of illnesses

www.sleepfoundation.org/site/c.huIXKjM0IxF/b. 2417141/k.2E30/The_National_Sleep_Foundation.htm

The National Sleep Foundation, which is committed to education, research, and advocacy on sleep. It includes a special component for children, "Sleep for Kids": www.sleepforkids.org/index.html

www.oflikeminds.com

The website of Moodletter, Inc., an organization committed to providing educational materials about mood and anxiety disorders

www.parenting.org

A parenting information website put out by Boystown, a nationally recognized social service agency for children with special treatment needs

Consumer Driven Support and Advocacy Organizations:

Alcoholics Anonymous (AA)
A.A. World Services, Inc.
P.O. Box 459
New York, NY 10163
(212) 870-3400
www.aa.org

Alcoholics Anonymous is an international, spiritually based association of people in recovery from alcoholism that uses a philosophy known as the "12 Steps" for recovery. It achieves its goal of helping people maintain sobriety through the use of group meetings and individual peer support. Documents of interest to adolescents include:

- *A message to Teenagers*
  www.aa.org/pdf/products/f-9_aMessagetoTeen agers1.pdf
- *Young People and AA*
  www.aa.org/pdf/products/p-4_youngpeopleandaa.pdf
- *Too Young?*
  www.aa.org/pdf/products/p-37_tooyoung.pdf

The National Alliance on Mental Illness (NAMI)
2107 Wilson Blvd., Suite 300
Arlington, VA 22201-3042
Main: (703) 524-7600
Fax: (703) 524-9094
TDD: (703) 516-7227
HelpLine: (800) 950-NAMI (6264)
Email: info@nami.org
www.nami.org

NAMI is the largest grassroots organization in the country for people with mental illness and their families.

175

Child & Adolescent Bipolar Foundation (CABF)
1000 Skokie Blvd., Suite 570
Wilmette, IL 60091
Email: cabf@bpkids.org
(847) 256-8525
www.bpkids.org/site/PageServer

The Depression and Bipolar Support Alliance (DBSA)
730 N. Franklin Street, Suite 501
Chicago, IL 60654-7225
Toll free: (800)826-3632
Fax: (312) 642-7243
www.dbsalliance.org/

The DBSA is a nationally run organization that aims to improve the lives of patients and families affected by mood disorders.

Narcotics Anonymous (NA)
Narcotics Anonymous World Services, Inc.
Main Office
P.O. Box 9999
Van Nuys, CA 91409
Telephone (818)773-9999
Fax (818) 700-0700
www.na.org

NA is an international, spiritually based association of people in recovery from drug abuse that uses the 12-Step model for recovery originally conceptualized by Alcoholics Anonymous. Regular group meetings and peer support (sponsorship) are at its foundation.

Under the section entitled, " Recovery literature," families might find these materials useful:

- Informational pamphlet #13: By Young Addicts, for Young Addicts
www.na.org/pdf/litfiles/us_english/IP/EN3113_2008.pdf
- Informational pamphlet #27: For the Parents or Guardians of Young People in NA
www.na.org/pdf/litfiles/us_english/IP/EN3127.pdf

Mental Health America (MHA)
Mental Health America
2000 N. Beauregard Street, 6th Floor
Alexandria, Virginia 22311
Main Switchboard: (703) 684-7722
Toll-free: (800) 969-6642
TTY: (800) 433-5959
Fax: (703) 684-5968
www.mentalhealthamerica.net

MHA is a nonprofit organization committed to promoting mental wellness throughout the United States. In addition to mental health advocacy, MHA can help find services and treatment on a local level as well as provide education on a variety of mental health topics.

Professional Organizations:

The American Academy of Child and Adolescent Psychiatry (AACAP)
3615 Wisconsin Avenue, N.W.
Washington, DC 20016-3007
Phone: (202) 966-7300
Fax: (202) 966-2891
www.aacap.org

The AACAP is the largest national organization for child and adolescent psychiatry in the United States It provides support, education, and advocacy to doctors and patients, as well as help finding a local child psychiatrist.

An important resource created by the AACAP is the Facts for Families Series, nearly 100 educational sheets on a variety of topics related to mental health and mental disorders:
www.aacap.org/cs/root/facts_for_families/facts_for_families_numerical_list

These sheets, selected from the website list of Facts for Families, may be especially useful for families with a mood disordered child:

- Teens: Alcohol and Other Drugs #3
- The Depressed Child #4
- Child Abuse—The Hidden Bruises #5
- Teen Suicide #10
- Children with Learning Disabilities #16
- The Child with a Long-Term Illness #19
- Psychiatric Medication for Children and Adolescents Part I: How Medications Are Used #21
- Normality #22
- When to Seek Help for Your Child #24
- Where to Find Help for Your Child #25
- Psychiatric Medication for Children and Adolescents Part II: Types of Medications #29
- Children's Sleep Problems #34
- Children and Firearms #37
- Bipolar Disorder (Manic-Depressive Illness) in Teens #38
- Children of Parents with Mental Illness #39
- Substance Abuse Treatment for Children and Adolescents: Questions to Ask #41
- The Continuum of Care #42
- Discipline #43
- The Anxious Child #47
- Schizophrenia in Children #49
- Psychiatric Medications for Children and Adolescents Part III: Questions to Ask #51

- Comprehensive Psychiatric Evaluation #52
- What Is Psychotherapy for Children and Adolescents? #53
- Understanding Violent Behavior in Children and Adolescents #55
- Normal Adolescent Development—Middle School and Early High School Years #57
- Normal Adolescent Development—Late High School Years and Beyond #58
- Foster Care #64
- Children's Threats: When Are They Serious? #65
- Helping Teenagers with Stress #66
- Posttraumatic Stress Disorder (PTSD) #70
- Self-Injury in Adolescents #73
- Obesity in Children and Teens #79
- Fighting and Biting #81
- Services in School for Children with Special Needs: What Parents Need to Know #83
- Talking to Kids About Mental Illnesses #84
- Psychotherapies for Children and Adolescents #86
- Preventing and Managing Medication-Related Weight Gain #94
- The Teen Brain: Behavior, Problem Solving, and Decision Making #95

The American Academy of Pediatrics (AAP)
141 Northwest Point Boulevard
Elk Grove Village, IL 60007-1098
Phone: (847) 434-4000
Fax: (847) 434-8000
www.aap.org

The AAP is the largest national organization for pediatricians and families. Like the AACAP, it has information on health topics, advocacy, and finding a doctor in the field.

Surviving

Government Run Organizations:

National Institute on Drug Abuse (NIDA)
National Institute on Drug Abuse
National Institutes of Health (NIH)
6001 Executive Boulevard, Room 5213
Bethesda, MD 20892-9561
Phone: (301) 443-1124
information@nida.nih.gov

NIDA is part of the NIH that conducts research and disseminates information on substance abuse. Websites of interest to children and teens include:
www.nida.nih.gov/MarijBroch/Marijteens.html
teens.drugabuse.gov/
teens.drugabuse.gov/mom/index.asp
teacher.scholastic.com/scholasticnews/indepth/headsup/

The National Institute of Mental Health (NIMH)
Science Writing, Press, and Dissemination Branch
6001 Executive Boulevard, Room 8184, MSC 9663
Bethesda, MD 20892-9663
Local: (301) 443-4513
Toll-free: (866) 615-6464
TTY: (301) 443-8431
TTY toll-free: (866) 415-8051
Fax: (301) 443-4279
www.nimh.nih.gov

The NIMH is the mental health organization of the National Institutes of Health (NIH), an agency of the U.S. Health and Human Services (HHS). The NIMH provides information about mental illnesses, promotes research studies, and disseminates the latest scientific findings in the field of mental health.

Substance Abuse and Mental Health Services Administration (SAMHSA)
SAMHSA's Health Information Network
P.O. Box 2345
Rockville, MD 20847-2345
Email: SHIN@samhsa.hhs.gov
Phone: (877) SAMHSA-7 ([877] 726-4727)
TTY: (800) 487-4889
Fax: (240) 221-4292
www.samhsa.gov
SAMHSA is an agency of the HHS that provides information on substance abuse and mental health. It also promotes research and advocacy on the treatment of these drug abuse and psychiatric disorders. A link is available to access treatment programs by geographic location:
www.csat.samhsa.gov

Several initiatives from SAMHSA that may be of interest to families living with depression or bipolar disorder include:

www.toosmarttostart.samhsa.gov/
Too Smart to Start, an initiative of SAMHSA to prevent underage drinking:

www.family.samhsa.gov
Family Guide, an initiative of SAMHSA that promotes mental health and seeks to prevent illegal drug abuse:

www.bblocks.samhsa.gov
Building Blocks for a Healthy Future, an initiative of SAMHSA to encourage communication with younger children and prevent substance abuse in later years:

mentalhealth.samhsa.gov/15plus/default.asp

15+ Make Time to Listen...Take Time to Talk, a campaign to encourage parents and children to spend at least 15 minutes a day talking and improve their relationship as well as build positive skills.

U.S. Food and Drug Administration (FDA)
5600 Fishers Lane
Rockville, MD 20857
(888) INFO-FDA ([888] 463-6332)
www.fda.gov

The FDA, an agency of the HHS, monitors medications, foods, and other products that may affect our health. It also has a special website for children to use: www.fda.gov/oc/opacom/kids/default.htm

Books

Your Child: Emotional, Behavioral, and Cognitive Development from Birth Through Preadolescence
By David Pruitt, MD, AACAP, Harper Collins, 2000

Your Adolescent: Emotional, Behavioral, and Cognitive Development from Early Adolescence Through the Teen Years
By David Pruitt, MD, AACAP, Harper Collins, 2000

Caring for Your Baby and Young Child: Birth to Age 5, 4th edition
By Steven P. Shelov, MD, MS, FAAP, Editor in Chief, and Robert E. Hannemann, MD, FAAP, American Academy of Pediatrics, 2004

An excellent primer on normal early childhood physical and emotional development as well as parenting.

Caring for Your School-Age Child: Ages 5 to 12
By Edward L. Schor, MD, FAAP, Editor in Chief, American Academy of Pediatrics, 2004

An excellent primer on normal physical and emotional development and parenting of school age children.

Caring for Your Teenager: The Complete and Authoritative Guide
Edited by Donald E. Greydanus, MD, FAAP, with Philip Bashe, American Academy of Pediatrics, 2006

An excellent primer on normal physical and emotional development and parenting teenagers.

Glossary

Addiction: According to the National Institute on Drug Abuse (NIDA), drug addiction is a brain disease characterized by compulsive drug seeking and use despite harmful consequences.

AIMS test: Also known as the Abnormal Involuntary Movement Scale. This is an examination done by a doctor or other trained health professional to test for tardive dyskinesia. It is a brief exam that is recorded onto a rating scale, and performed every few months to monitor for the development of tardive dyskinesia.

Alternative treatment: The use of non-traditional treatments instead of those typically prescribed in Western medicine. An example would be the use of Chinese herbs to treat depression.

Akathisia: A feeling of inner restlessness often caused by medications such as antipsychotics or antidepressants. Outer signs of akathisia include motor restlessness such as fidgetiness.

Anticholinergic medications: A family of medications acting upon the neurotransmitter, acetylcholine, which helps reverse some of the side effects such as acute muscle spasms and restlessness caused by psychotropic medications. A commonly used anticholinergic medications is benztropine (trade name Cogentin).

Anticonvulsants: Medications used to treat or prevent seizures. This family of medications often has utility in the treatment of BPD for mood stabilization (see Table 18).

Antipsychotics: Medications used to treat psychosis (hallucinations, delusions, or other distortions in the perception of reality).

Augmentation: The addition of a second medication to a primary one, in order to boost the effects of the first medication. Common augmentation agents for depression include lithium, thyroid hormone, and bupropion. Often a smaller dose of the augmentation agent is used to assist the primary medication.

Autism: Also known as autistic disorder in the *DSM*. Autism is a neurodevelopmental disorder that begins in infancy and early childhood that is characterized by profound deficits in social functioning and communication, restricted interests, and/or repetitive behaviors.

Benzodiazepines: A class of medications used to treat anxiety, seizures, insomnia, or alcohol withdrawal. These medicines act upon a set of neurotransmitters that cause calming and sedation.

Biogenic amines: Three neurotransmitters traditionally associated with mood and anxiety disorders. These include dopamine, norepinephrine, and serotonin. Imbalances of other neurotransmitters have since been found to play a role in disorders of mood and anxiety, however, the biogenic amines continue to be of central importance in the biochemistry of mood disorders.

Borderline Personality Disorder: (see Table 14) This disorder is characterized by self-injurious behavior, along with distortions in self image, relationships with others, black and white thinking, fears of abandonment, and other features.

Comorbid conditions: The presence of two or more psychiatric disorders in the same individual. An example would be having ADHD and depression.

Complementary treatment: The use of non-traditional treatments along with typical treatments prescribed in Western medicine. An example would be the use of yoga with medications for anxiety.

Compliance: The extent to which treatment recommendations are followed by a patient.

Cyclothymia: Also referred to as "cyclothymic disorder." According to the *DSM*, in children and adolescents cyclothymic disorder is diagnosed when a year or more of numerous periods of hypomanic and depressive symptoms, along with other criteria are observed (see Table 5). It is used in cases where BPD or MDD is difficult to determine because the fluctuations of mood are often too rapid, too short in duration, or too mild in severity to fit the usual definition of these disorders.

Dependence: Continued need to use a drug without which a physical or psychological reaction would occur. Often a pattern of seeking the drug has been established.

Discontinuation syndrome: An unpleasant bodily experience occurring within a few days to weeks of abruptly stopping a medication or missing doses, especially the SSRIs or other antidepressants. The experience often includes flu-like symptoms such as headache, dizziness, nausea, and other neurologic or gastrointestinal complaints, as well as possible mood and anxiety symptoms. The discontinuation syndrome seems to occur more frequently when medications that are metabolized more quickly in the body (e.g., paroxetine) are stopped versus medicines that are metabolized more slowly (e.g., fluoxetine). The discontinuation syndrome is generally considered mild or inconvenient, and subsides on its own. It can be avoided or minimized by gradual tapering of the medicine over a few days to weeks.

Dopamine: Neurotransmitter associated with pleasure seeking and reward, motor functions in the body (movement), attention and organizational skills. An imbalance in dopamine is associated with hallucinations.

Dual diagnosis: The situation of having both a psychiatric disorder such as a mood disorder or schizophrenia and a substance abuse disorder.

Dysthymic disorder: Also known as "dysthymia." According to the *DSM*, dysthymic disorder is diagnosed in children and adolescents when a depressed or irritable mood is observed almost all the time for a year or more, and at least two symptoms drawing from the list for an MDE, as well as other features are also noted (see Table 8).

Dystonia: Also known as a dystonic reaction. The sudden or gradual development of uncomfortable and possibly painful spasms of muscle groups in the neck, eyes, extremities, or muscles involved in speech and breathing. The problem develops within a few hours or days after a medication, especially an antipsychotic is started or increased

in dose. Dystonia often responds to anticholinergic medications, or to removal of the offending agent.

Endogenous opiates: Naturally occurring chemicals in the body that are released by pain or stress, that result in numbing or decreased perception of pain.

Hypersomnia: Sleeping in excess of what is normally expected for one's age. An example would be a depressed teenager sleeping 15 hours a day instead of 8 or 9.

Hypomania: Behavior that would fit the criteria for a hypomanic episode. A hypomanic episode is described in the *DSM* as a period of elevated or irritable mood for 4 days or more, along with other criteria (see Table 3).

IEP: Also known as an Individual Educational Plan. This is a document created by educators for a child with special educational needs that may call for smaller class size, additional instruction in certain subjects such as math or reading, or additional services such as counseling and/or special therapies such as speech or handwriting (occupational therapy). Parental input is usually invited in the creation of an IEP.

Insomnia: Difficulty in falling asleep or staying asleep. The problem can occur early at night where the inability to fall asleep is noted, in the middle of the night with an awakening and inability to fall back asleep, or too early in the morning where an awakening occurs well before scheduled wake up time and the inability to fall back asleep is noted.

Manic switch: A situation where a patient with BPD becomes suddenly manic during a depressed episode. Antidepressants sometimes cause manic switches in vulnerable bipolar patients, especially those who are not on mood stabilizers.

Mood Disorders: Any of several types of depression or bipolar disorders that are defined in the Diagnostic and Statistical Manual (DSM).

Neuroimaging tests: Commonly known as "brain scans," these include computer tomography (CT or CAT scans), magnetic resonance imaging (MRIs), and other tests looking at the structure of the brain or its function.

Neuroleptic malignant syndrome: Known commonly as "NMS." This is a life-threatening, but rare condition brought on by antipsychotic use. It requires hospital care, usually in the intensive care unit, and includes symptoms of fever, severe muscle rigidity, and other abnormalities of the nervous system.

Norepinephrine: A neurotransmitter involved with attention, associated with the "fight or flight" response that acts upon heart rate and blood pressure, and is involved with arousal and wakefulness.

Placebo: A pill used in research which resembles the study drug, but is actually a "dummy" or "sugar" pill that contains no active drug. The use of a placebo is important in research because it helps demonstrate if the study drug is effective in people who are taking the drug versus people who are not taking it, but think they are taking it. Giving a placebo to a comparison subject is considered better in research than giving no pill, because it controls for other factors such as the psychological benefit of taking a pill.

Play therapy: Includes a range of therapeutic approaches using toys or props. Play is children's way of mastering things in the world that include completing tasks, processing ideas, solving problems, and developing relationships needed for their growth and development, and also feeling safe.

Post-traumatic stress disorder: Also known as "PTSD." This is a *DSM* disorder that is characterized by groups of symptoms that include hyperarousal, avoidance, and reexperiencing an event after having been exposed to a life-threatening or harmful event. More details about PTSD are described in Table 11.

Prodromal stage: A period of time before diagnosis of an illness such as bipolar disorder or a psychotic disorder, when symptoms exist but are much more subtle and not yet causing disability. The period can exist for months or years before the illness fully presents.

Prophylaxis: The use of medication to prevent the occurrence of an episode of illness. An example would be the use of a mood stabilizer in a patient with BPD to prevent manic episodes.

Psychoeducation: Patient education through written materials, other media, or discussion on topics relevant to psychiatric illness and treatment.

Psychostimulants: Also known as "stimulants." Medications that increase the brain's alertness, hence the name. Two major categories of psychostimulants include methylphenidate and amphetamine. This group of medications is used to treat ADHD as well as a problem with wakefulness known as narcolepsy.

Psychotropic medications: Medications which act specifically and primarily upon the brain, in contrast to other parts of the body, as in the case of asthma medications acting upon the lungs (but not the brain).

Receptor: A structure on the end of a receiving nerve cell into which a traveling neurotransmitter such as serotonin can attach. Once a neurotransmitter has attached to a receptor, further changes in the chemical activity of the cell may occur. Different chemical activities among antidepressants as well as the side effects experienced are often defined by the receptors that they act upon.

Recurrence: A situation where a new episode of depression occurs after a first episode resolves, usually after 2 months or more of improvement.

Relapse: A situation where the symptoms of depression return within a short time of improvement, usually between 2 weeks and 2 months of the improvement.

Remission: Reduction or resolution of depressive symptoms in the early stages of the illness, between 2 weeks and 2 months.

Resilience: The ability for some children to adapt or succeed despite adversity.

Response: Reduction or resolution of psychiatric symptoms. A partial response to treatment during a depressive or manic episode is a reduced number of symptom criteria, while a full response results in a complete resolution of symptoms (also known as remission).

Serotonin: A neurotransmitter associated with control of mood, appetite, memory, and sleep. Deficiencies in serotonin appear to cause depression and anxiety.

Serotonin syndrome: A situation created by taking an excess of medications that boosts serotonin activity in the body. It includes sweating, tremor, agitation, various neurologic symptoms like increased muscle reactivity, and mental confusion. The most serious version of serotonin syndrome can be life-threatening and can occur with the combination of an MAOI and an SSRI.

Sleep diary: A written record describing several days' worth of sleep and wake times at night, daytime naps, and total number of hours of sleep every day. The sleep diary helps your doctor understand how much or how little your child is sleeping and could give more information about possible sleep disorders or problems in the sleeping routine.

Sleep-wake cycle: The biological pattern that occurs every 24 hours of sleep followed by wakefulness.

Substance abuse: Repeated use of illicit drugs that leads to negative consequences.

Subtherapeutic dose: An amount of medication below what is needed to be effective in treating the symptoms for which it is prescribed. The amount of medication that is effective is called the therapeutic dose or therapeutic window (if a range of doses is therapeutic).

Suicidality: Suicidal thoughts, actions such as suicide attempts, or other harmful behaviors that could lead to suicide.

Tardive dyskinesia: A permanent movement disorder that occurs months to years after using antipsychotic medications. These include movements in the face and mouth such as involuntary grimacing, tongue thrusting or chewing, and in the body such as swaying of the torso or hips, and repetitive movements of the fingers. The risk for tardive dyskinesia increases the longer someone is taking antipsychotic medications, and at higher doses. The newer antipsychotics appear to cause tardive dyskinesia less often than the older ones, although all antipsychotics carry risk

for the developing the disorder with long term use. The severity of tardive dyskinesia can be lessened at times with a switch or reduction in antipsychotic medications. Over time, the disorder may increase or subside in intensity, and is more of nuisance and a cosmetic issue than a threat to general health.

Tolerance: The need for higher doses of a medication to have the same effect after prolonged use.

Tourette's Disorder: A childhood onset disorder characterized by motor and vocal tics. Tics are a type of sudden, repetitive movements or vocal sounds.

Treatment plan: A written document in the medical record or a conceptual outline used by the clinician that names important goals in a child's psychiatric treatment. Often, a time frame in which the goals are to be achieved is named in the treatment plan along with examples that would illustrate reduction or improvement in the symptoms for which treatment is sought in the first place.

Withdrawal: A physical or psychological reaction that occurs when a drug of abuse is discontinued. Craving or drug seeking is generally associated with withdrawal.

Index

Italicized page locators indicate a table are noted with a *t*

Index

Index